DELAYED PRECONDITIONING AND ADAPTIVE CARDIOPROTECTION

Developments in
Cardiovascular Medicine

VOLUME 207

The titles published in this series are listed at the end of this volume.

Delayed Preconditioning and Adaptive Cardioprotection

edited by

G. F. BAXTER

The Hatter Institute for Cardiovascular Studies,
University College London Medical School, London, U.K.

and

D. M. YELLON

The Hatter Institute for Cardiovascular Studies,
University College London Medical School, London, U.K.

KLUWER ACADEMIC PUBLISHERS

DORDRECHT / BOSTON / LONDON

A C.I.P. Catalogue record for this book is available from the Library of Congress.

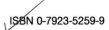
ISBN 0-7923-5259-9

Published by Kluwer Academic Publishers,
P.O. Box 17, 3300 AA Dordrecht, The Netherlands.

Sold and distributed in North, Central and South America
by Kluwer Academic Publishers,
101 Philip Drive, Norwell, MA 02061, U.S.A.

In all other countries, sold and distributed
by Kluwer Academic Publishers,
P.O. Box 322, 3300 AH Dordrecht, The Netherlands.

Printed on acid-free paper

Cover drawing by Dr Robert Bell

Contents

Preface

The formal recognition by Charles Murry, Robert Jennings and Keith Reimer in 1986 that myocardium possesses the ability to adapt rapidly to transient ischaemic stress proved to be the impetus for a remarkable explosion in experimental and clinical cardiology research. Many who had previously devoted their valuable time to the investigation of stategies for protection of the ischaemic myocardium were so impressed by the potency of this endogenous cardioprotective response that they opted to examine the phenomenon of myocardial preconditioning in their own laboratories. The results of these investigations have yielded an enormous literature during the last decade. The majority of this work has been devoted to investigating the characteristics and molecular mechanisms of what is now known as the classic preconditioning response originally described by Murry, Jennings and Reimer.

In 1993, two reports heralded the recognition of another aspect of myocardial adaptation to ischaemia, namely a delayed preconditioning response which we termed the "second window" of protection. This phenomenon has proved to be of increasing interest because it represents a further feature of the heart's ability to adapt to stressful stimuli. During the last five years, a number of studies have extended the definitions of delayed preconditioning by describing its ability to protect against a variety of ischaemia-reperfusion pathologies. Understanding of the potential triggers, cell signalling pathways and downstream mediators of this sub-acute form of adaptive cardioprotection has advanced considerably in this period.

In view of a burgeoning literature, reflecting the interest in delayed preconditioning and related adaptive cardioprotective strategies, we felt it timely to compile a series of state-of-the-art reviews by those people who have made significant contributions to the advance of this field. The chapters contained in this book describe a very rapid advance in delayed preconditioning reseach, from its molecular basis to potential clinical relevance. All of the authors, who are internationally recognised experts, discuss the various aspects of this subject in detail and their contributions have permitted us to produce what we hope is a comprehensive and up-to-date text. Accordingly, we believe that the contents of this book provide valuable insights into the processes that occur in the myocardium under stress, extend our understanding of these adaptive phenomena and point to new approaches which may be exploitable in the search for effective cardioprotective strategies. We hope that this compilation will provide an authoritative and informative overview for researchers engaged in the exploration of this fascinating area but we leave our readers to adjudicate on this matter for themselves.

Gary F Baxter
Derek M Yellon   London 1998

Acknowledgments

The preparation of this book would not have been possible without the help of many people. The contributors to the volume must receive our special thanks. We are aware of the considerable time and effort that each has spent in preparing chapters, in spite of other pressures and diversions that continually present. We credit the authors with the production of chapters that combine both depth of treatment and critical approach. As editors, we have regarded ourselves as informed facilitators for the production of a text that we hope is reasonably uniform in style, eschews unnecessary jargon and pays some attention to the niceties of prose composition. Our job has been eased by our publishers. Nettie Dekker and Evelien Bakker at Kluwer Academic Publishers provided practical assistance, gentle encouragement and advice, from inception to production, which have been greatly appreciated. Finally, on a personal note, our greatest debt of gratitude is owed to two people behind the scenes, John and Luci, whose continued patience and understanding were necessary for us to indulge in our pursuit of academic gratification.

Gary F Baxter
Derek M Yellon

London 1998

Contributors

G F Baxter The Hatter Institute for Cardiovascular Studies, Division of Cardiology, University College London Hospital & Medical School, Grafton Way, London WC1E 6DB, UK

P Beauchamp Service de Pharmacologie, Hopital de Bois Guillaume, CHU, 76031 Rouen Cedex, France

R Bolli Division of Cardiology, University of Louisville, ACB Third Floor, 550 South Jackson Street, Louisville, Kentucky 40292, USA

R W Currie Department of Anatomy and Neurobiology, Dalhousie University, Sir Charles Tupper Building, Halifax, Nova Scotia B3H 4H7, Canada

A Dana The Hatter Institute for Cardiovascular Studies, Division of Cardiology, University College London Hospital & Medical School, Grafton Way, London WC1E 6DB, UK

D K Das Cardiovascular Division, Department of Surgery, University of Conneticut School of Medicine, 263 Farmington Avenue, Farmington, Conneticut 06030-1110, USA

B Dawn Division of Cardiology, University of Louisville, ACB Third Floor, 550 South Jackson Street, Louisville, Kentucky 40292, USA

D Ferrini Fondazione Cardiologica Myriam Zito Sacco, Piazza Fratelli Ruffini 6, 47100 Forli, Italy

M Galvani Fondazione Cardiologica Myriam Zito Sacco, Piazza Fratelli Ruffini 6, 47100 Forli, Italy

G J Gross Department of Pharmacology and Toxicology, Medical College of Wisconsin, 8701 Watertown Plank Road, Milwaukie, Wisconsin 53226, USA

M Hori First Department of Medicine, Osaka University Medical School, 2-2 Yamada-oka, Suita, Osaka 565, Japan

N Kaeffer Service de Pharmacologie, Hopital de Bois Guillaume, CHU, 76031 Rouen Cedex, France

T Kuzuya First Department of Medicine, Osaka University Medical School, 2-2 Yamada-oka, Suita, Osaka 565, Japan

L V Mayne The Trafford Centre for Medical Research, University of Sussex, Falmer, Brighton BN1 9RY, UK

F Ottani Fondazione Cardiologica Myriam Zito Sacco, Piazza Fratelli Ruffini 6, 47100 Forli, Italy

J R Parratt Department of Physiology and Pharmacology, University of Strathclyde, Glasgow G1 1XW, UK

P Ping Division of Cardiology, University of Louisville, ACB Third Floor, 550 South Jackson Street, Louisville, Kentucky 40292, USA

J-C L Plumier Department of Anatomy and Neurobiology, Dalhousie University, Sir Charles Tupper Building, Halifax, Nova Scotia B3H 4H7, Canada

Y Qiu Division of Cardiology, University of Louisville, ACB Third Floor, 550 South Jackson Street, Louisville, Kentucky 40292, USA

V Richard Service de Pharmacologie, Hopital de Bois Guillaume, CHU, 76031 Rouen Cedex, France

H Takano Division of Cardiology, University of Louisville, ACB Third Floor, 550 South Jackson Street, Louisville, Kentucky 40292, USA

X-L Tang Division of Cardiology, University of Louisville, ACB Third Floor, 550 South Jackson Street, Louisville, Kentucky 40292, USA

C Thuillez Service de Pharmacologie, Hopital de Bois Guillaume, CHU, 76031 Rouen Cedex, France

A Vegh Department of Pharmacology, Albert Szent-Gyorgyi Medical University, P O Box 115, 6701 Szeged, Hungary

N Yamashita First Department of Medicine, Osaka University Medical School, 2-2 Yamada-oka, Suita, Osaka 565, Japan

D M Yellon The Hatter Institute for Cardiovascular Studies, Division of Cardiology, University College London Hospital & Medical School, Grafton Way, London WC1E 6DB, UK

J Zhang Division of Cardiology, University of Louisville, ACB Third Floor, 550 South Jackson Street, Louisville, Kentucky 40292, USA

1

Delayed Preconditioning Against Lethal Ischaemic Injury

G F Baxter and D M Yellon

1. Introduction

Two experimental studies were published in 1993 describing the ability of myocardium to acquire tolerance to lethal ischaemic injury 24 hours following transient sublethal periods of ischaemia [1, 2]. These two studies initiated an area of research on ischaemic preconditioning of myocardium which has developed considerably in the last five years. This form of preconditioning, known variously as "delayed preconditioning", "late preconditioning", the "second window of protection" or the "second window of preconditioning", is clearly a form of endogenous protection which shares many features in common with other procedures and interventions (described before and after 1993) that enhance tissue tolerance to ischaemic stress in a sub-acute manner. Several treatments that are able to induce this pattern of protection are described elsewhere in this volume and these include heat stress (chapter 7), endotoxin and its derivatives (chapter 9), and adenosine analogues (chapter 10). In this chapter, we will review the background to the discovery of delayed preconditioning, the characteristics of this phenomenon and possible mechanisms. We will concentrate particularly on the direct cytoprotective properties of delayed preconditioning i.e. the ability of delayed preconditioning to protect myocardium against lethal ischaemia-reperfusion injury in vivo and in vitro.

2. Background

Brief periods of ischaemia induce two forms of adaptation in myocardium that are associated with the acquisition of tolerance to subsequent ischaemic episodes (see figure 1). An acutely manifested form of adaptation was described by Murry, Jennings and Reimer [3] who introduced the term "preconditioning" into the lexicon of experimental cardiology in their seminal study. This early form of preconditioning, now often referred to as "classic preconditioning" is observed immediately following brief sublethal ischaemia and confers a marked slowing of the progression of irreversible ischaemic injury during subsequent ischaemia. This delay in the onset of irreversible tissue injury and cell death results in limitation of infarct size [3]. The limitation of tissue injury by classic preconditioning is a potent effect. Additionally, classic preconditioning in some species confers protection against the severe ventricular rhythm disturbances that occur during subsequent ischaemia and reperfusion [4, 5]. Although the limitation of tissue injury may result in improved post-ischaemic contractile recovery of myocardium, classic preconditioning does not appear to afford protection against the phenomenon of myocardial stunning i.e. depressed contractile recovery in the absence of irreversible tissue injury [6]. One of the most distinctive features of classic preconditioning is that the protection afforded by antecedent ischaemia wanes rapidly. In most models, no protection against either infarction or arrhythmias is observed when the interval between preconditioning and the subsequent ischaemic insult is extended beyond two hours. Thus, while classic preconditioning affords very potent protection, its effect is short-lived.

We now know that an additional form of adaptation is simulated by similar ischaemic preconditioning stimuli. A delayed form of adaptation is manifested sub-acutely around 24 hours following preconditioning and is observed as protection against a variety of ischaemic pathologies. These include irreversible tissue and cell injury both in vivo and in vitro which are the focus of this chapter. In addition, delayed preconditioning attenuates myocardial stunning (chapter 2), post-ischaemic vascular endothelial dysfunction (chapter 3) and ventricular arrhythmias during ischaemia and reperfusion (chapter 4).

3. Discovery of Delayed Preconditioning

The formal recognition that ischaemic preconditioning induces a biphasic pattern of protection against subsequent lethal ischaemic injury was made independently in our laboratory [1] and in Osaka [2]. Both groups were investigating the changes occurring in the transcription of stress protein or anti-oxidant genes in response to sublethal ischaemia. In our laboratory, recognition of a "second window of preconditioning"

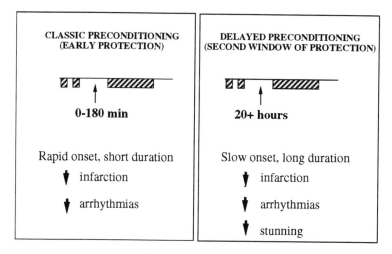

Figure 1. Preconditioning myocardium with one or more brief periods of ischaemia results in marked protection against a subsequent period of ischaemia. Protection is observed in two distinct phases. Early protection ("classic" preconditioning) is apparent immediately but disappears within 2-3 hours. A subsequent delayed period of protection can be observed beyond 20 hours after preconditioning ("second window of protection").

arose from work directed towards investigating the mechanisms of sub-acute adaptation of myocardium following whole body hyperthermia (heat stress). Several groups have shown that 24 hours following heat stress, hearts from rats and rabbits display enhanced tolerance to the consequences of subsequent ischaemia-repefusion (see chapter 7 for a full account). This acquired tolerance to ischaemia-reperfusion as part of the heat stress response, is associated with the expression of several proteins, including an inducible form of the 70 kDa heat stress protein (HSP70i). There had been reports that sublethal myocardial ischaemia itself could also increase the expression of HSP70i in myocardium [7, 8]) and this seemed to offer a more pathophysiologically relevant method of inducing HSP70i expression in the heart. The hypothesis under investigation was that if HSP70i expression in the myocardium was induced by transient ischaemia, and was per se a cytoprotective protein, then brief transient ischaemia (ischaemic preconditioning) should, several hours later when tissue HSP70i levels were raised, also confer protection against a subsequent sustained ischaemic insult. To examine this hypothesis an experiment was conducted using a rabbit model of preconditioning with four 5 minute coronary artery occlusions and subsequent recovery [1]. Twenty four hours following this preconditioning stimulus, the animals were subjected to a 30 minute period of coronary occlusion and infarct size was determined after 120

Table 1. Delayed preconditioning against experimental myocardial infarction in vivo

Species	PC protocol	Index ischaemia	Interval	I/R reduction	Reference
Dog	4x5 min	90 min	24 h	46% reduction	Kuzuya [2]
Dog	4x5 min	90 min	24 h	50% reduction	Node [26]
Rabbit	4x5 min	30 min	24 h	44% reduction	Marber [1]
Rabbit	4x5 min	30 min	24 h	39% reduction	Baxter [10]
Rabbit	4x5 min	30 min	24, 48, 72 h	35, 53, 57% reduction	Baxter [11]
Rabbit	1, 2 or 4x5	30 min	48 h	44, 38, 45% reduction	Baxter [11]
Rabbit	4x5 min	30 min	24 h	35% reduction	Baxter [12]
Rabbit	4x5 min	30 min	24 h	32% reduction	Yang [18]
Rabbit	4x5 min	30 min	48 h	55% reduction	Imagawa [13]
Rabbit	4x5 min	30 min	48 h	58% reduction	Imagawa [14]
Rabbit	4x5 min	30 min	24 h	50% reduction	Qiu [19]
Rabbit	4x5 min	30 min	24 h	50% reduction	Takano [20]
Rabbit	4x5 min	30 min	24 h	71% reduction	Okubo [15]
Rabbit	4x5 min	30 min	24 h	41% reduction	Li [16]

Table 1 (continued).

Species	PC protocol	Index ischaemia	Interval	I/R reduction	Reference
Rabbit	4x5 min	30 min	24 h	40% reduction	Li [17]
Rabbit	4x5 min	30 min	24 h	no reduction	Tanaka [21]
Rabbit	4x5 min	30 min	24 h	27% reduction with TTC no reduction with histology	Miki [22]
Pig	4x5 min	60 min	24 h	15% reduction (NS)	Strasser [31]
Pig*	10x2 min 25x2 min	40 min 40 min	24 h 24 h	26% reduction (NS) 14% reduction (NS)	Qiu [32]
Pig	4x5 min	40 min	24 h	53% reduction	Muller [33]
Rat	2x5 min	30 min	24 h	34% reduction	Yamashita [27]
Rat	1x2 + 2x5 min	20 min	24 h	27% reduction	Kaeffer [28]
Rat	3x3 min 15 min	45 min 45 min	24 h 24 h	no reduction no reduction	Jagasia [29]

Preconditioning (PC) protocols and index ischaemia protocols indicate duration of coronary artery occlusion.* indicates studies conducted in conscious (non-anaesthetised) animals. I/R reduction is relative reduction in infarct size determined by triphenyltetrazolium chloride (TTC) macrochemistry unless otherwise stated. NS = statistically non significant ($p > 0.05$). All other I/R reductions were reported to be statistically significant ($p < 0.05$).

minutes reperfusion using triphenyltetrazolium macrochemical staining. Risk volume was determined with a fluorescent microsphere exclusion technique. The percentage of infarcted myocardium within the risk zone (% I/R) was reduced from 52% to 29%, representing a 44% relative reduction in infarct size. This protection was very similar to the protection observed in a separate group of animals following prior heat stress where there was a 42% reduction in I/R. Twenty four hours following both ischaemic preconditioning and prior heat stress, HSP70i was also shown to be elevated several-fold. In addition, the mitochondrial stress protein HSP60 was also shown to be elevated by ischaemic preconditioning but to a lesser degree, and was not elevated by heat stress.

At the same time, workers led by Kuzuya in Osaka were examining the hypothesis that repetitive brief ischaemia with reperfusion induced alterations in the endogenous anti-oxidant activity of the post-ischaemic myocardium and that these might confer enhanced tolerance to subsequent ischaemia (see chapter 8 for a fuller account). Their observation of delayed preconditoning was contained in two related papers. Hoshida et al. [9] initially showed that the myocardial content of manganese superoxide dismutase (Mn-SOD) increased gradually in the ischaemic and non-ischaemic zones over 72 hours following ischaemic preconditioning. This initial work was followed by a report from the same group describing the time course of infarct limitation between 3 and 24 hours after preconditioning [2]. Differences in ischaemic myocardial blood flow were not observed over the time course of these experiments suggesting a direct cardioprotective mechanism, independent of collateral vessel recruitment.

4. Characteristics of Delayed Preconditioning Against Infarction

Species and Experimental Determinants

Following the initial reports, delayed preconditioning against infarction has been observed in every species examined so far (see Table 1). By far the majority of studies have been conducted in rabbit myocardium. The delayed anti-infarct effect in the rabbit has been confirmed in further open-chest rabbit studies [10-17] and also in chronically-instrumented conscious rabbits [18-20]. In most rabbit studies, several cycles of preconditioning have been adopted with an index ischaemic insult of 30 minutes. With this protocol, relative reduction in I/R is around 45%.

In a study undertaken to confirm delayed preconditioning against infarction in the rabbit, Tanaka et al. [21] demonstrated the protective effects of classic preconditioning in this model (a 72% reduction in infarct size), but no protection was observed 24 or 48 hours later. Miki et al. [22] have recently reported that in conscious rabbits, preconditioning induced a delayed modest reduction in infarct size, visualised by tetrazolium macrochemistry. However, they could detect no limitation of infarction using histological evaluation. The reason for this discordancy is not clear. This group proposed previously that exogenously administered SOD could cause false-positive staining with tetrazolium [23] and have suggested that upregulation of endogenous SOD by preconditioning may account for an artefactual limitation of infarct size by delayed preconditioning. However, other groups who have specifically examined the question of SOD influence on tetrazolium macrochemistry have found no evidence that SOD artefactually influences tetrazolium staining [24, 25]. Reasons for the absence of protection in some studies of delayed preconditoning therefore remain unclear but the detection of delayed preconditioning may be markedly influenced by technical factors such as differences in surgical preparation, model-dependent factors such as anaesthesia and other drug influences, and biological factors such as general condition, stress state of the animals and the variability of inflammatory responses.

In the dog, following the initial report [2], a subsequent study has been reported describing limitation of infarction by delayed preconditioning [26]. The rat is another species in which a second window of protection has been described. Recently, Yamashita et al. [27] have shown that preconditioning with two 3 minute coronary occlusions, each separated by 5 minute reperfusion, protected against a 30 minute occlusion 24 hours later. I/R was reduced from 62% in sham operated animals to 41% in preconditioned animals. An essentially similar pattern of protection was reported in the rat by Kaeffer [28] (see also chapter 3). However, a failure to observe delayed preconditionining against infarction in the rat has been reported by Jagasia et al. [29]. It is worth noting here that possibly the first delayed preconditioning study was in the rat examining reperfusion-induced arrhythmias. The interval between the first coronary occlusion and the second (or index) coronary occlusion was extended to 24 hours at which time no reduction in arryhthmia incidence or severity was seen [30].

Three studies have been undertaken in pig myocardium. Two studies did not observe statistically significant limitation of infarction 24 hours later. In the first of these studies, Strasser et al. [31] reported that four 5 minute cycles of ischaemia failed to elicit protection against a sustained 60 minute coronary occlusion 24 hours later (I/R was 71% in controls v 60% in preconditoned). We feel it very likely that the duration of this sustained ischaemic insult in a non-collateralised species may have been too severe to permit demonstration of a protective effect. A further study in the pig was more carefully designed to examine the possibility of a second window of protection [32]. Qiu et al. examined the effects of repeated brief coronary occlusions (10 x 2 minute) in conscious pigs 24 hours before a 40 minute occlusion. In the preconditioned group a 26% relative reduction in I/R was observed (I/R 45% v 33%) but this was not statistically significant. A further group of animals preconditioned with 25 x 2 minute occlusions did not display further enhancement of ischaemic tolerance at 24 hours and these workers concluded that a second window of protection against infarction does not occur in the pig. However, the modest limitation of infarct size in this study encouraged us to think that the pig is capable of exhibiting delayed preconditioning under favourable circumstances, i.e. with an ideal preconditioning stimulus, the correct time point of intervention, limitation of surgical trauma and psychological stress, and with a milder index ischaemic insult. We have addressed this possibility in a collaborative study with Muller and colleagues in Cape Town [33]. Under anaesthesia, pigs underwent coronary catheterisation through a carotid incision and were preconditioned by four 5 minute balloon inflations in the mid-left anterior descending coronary artery (LAD) region. The animals were allowed to recover from this minor surgical procedure. Twenty to 24 hours later, they were reanaesthetised with isoflurane and subjected to a 40 minute occlusion of the LAD. The results are shown in figure 2. Preconditioning on the previous day resulted in significant limitation of infarct size (30% in controls vs 14% in preconditioned animals) suggesting that the pig is indeed capable of exhibiting delayed preconditioning against infarction. It should be noted that the duration of index ischaemia was identical to that used by Qiu et al. [32] but in our open-chest model resulted in a 30% infarct-to-risk ratio whereas Qiu et al. reported a 45% infarct-to-risk ratio in conscious pigs (see figure 2). It is likely that cardiac temperature was a major determinant of this difference.

Natural History of Protection in Rabbit Myocardium

The delayed onset of the second window of protection, originally described in the study of Kuzuya et al. (1993) [2], suggested that it was likely to be of greater duration than classic preconditioning protection. We demonstrated that the delayed anti-infarct effect of preconditioning in the rabbit extends over a period of 3 days [11]. Interestingly, the magnitude of the infarct-limiting effect in the rabbit increases as the interval between preconditioning and acute myocardial infarction is extended beyond 24 hours and is maximal 48-72 hours after preconditioning. By 96 hours after preconditioning, however, no protection against infarction is seen. With regard to other endpoints, an investigation of the time course of rapid pacing-induced delayed protection against arrhythmias in dogs , found that protection against fibrillation (and hence mortality) was almost completely lost by 48 hours [34] (see also chapter 4). However, there was evidence that even

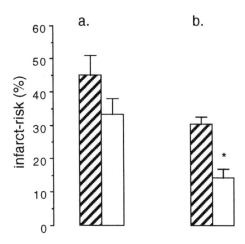

Figure 2. Delayed preconditioning against infarction in pig myocardium. Hatched bars, control animals; open bars, preconditioned animals. Panel a. shows the infarct size observed in a study by Qiu et al. [32]. Chronically instrumented pigs were preconditioned in the conscious state with ten 2 minute coronary occlusions and then 24 hours later subjected to a 40 minute coronary occlusion, also in the conscious state. A 26% reduction in infarct size was observed in the preconditioned group relative to the control group but this was not statistically significant. Panel b. shows the results of a similar study conducted by Muller et al. [33]. Pigs were preconditioned while anaesthetised by four 5 minute PTCA ballon inflations. After 24 hours they were subjected to an open-chest 40 minute coronary occlusion. Preconditioned animals showed a significant 50% reduction in infarct size relative to controls. Note that the control infarct size is smaller than that observed in panel a., probably reflecting the influences of anaesthesia and reduced body temperature. This study suggests that with a relatively mild ischaemic insult and an appropriate preconditioning stimulus, delayed preconditioning against infarction can be observed in the pig. * $P < 0.01$.

72 hours later, some attenuation of parameters such as electrical inhomogeneity was present. With regard to the time course of the second window against myocardial stunning in the pig, Sun et al. initially reported that the anti-stunning effect could be renewed by preconditioning again after 24 hours so that protection was seen 48 hours after the first stunning protocol [35] . No protection was observed after a 10 day interval between the preconditioning protocol and the subsequent stunning protocol. More recently, this group has examined the time course of this delayed anti-stunning phenomenon more specifically [36]. They have shown that the systolic wall thickening deficit was reduced when the second stunning protocol was induced 12 hours, 24 hours and 72 hours after the first stunning protocol but no protection was observed 6 days after preconditioning (see chapter 2).

Thus the experimental evidence suggests that the time courses of delayed preconditioning against infarction in the rabbit and delayed preconditioning against stunning in the pig are rather similar.

An interesting characteristic of delayed preconditioning against infarction is the threshold of preconditioning ischaemia required to trigger the cellular adaptation. In classic preconditioning against infarction, it seems that the response may not be dose-dependent; multiple short cycles of preconditioning ischaemia do not confer greater protection than a single 5 minute period [37]. In contrast, the delayed myocardial protection that occurs 24 hours after whole body heat stress appears to be related to the severity of the initiating trigger, i.e. the degree of protection correlates with the maximal core temperature achieved during heat stress [39]. We undertook a study in rabbits to assess the threshold for eliciting delayed preconditioning against infarction and the possibility that the degree of protection elicited was related to the number of preceding preconditioning coronary occlusions [11]. A surprising finding was that a single 5 minute coronary occlusion was as effective as four 5 minute occlusions in inducing delayed protection 48 hours later. This result implies a sharp threshold of initiation for the adaptive response resulting in delayed preconditioning, unlike heat shock which induces delayed cardioprotection in a manner that is apparently related to the severity of the priming stimulus [38].

We believe that delayed preconditioning against lethal ischaemic injury is an important protective response in myocardium. The pattern of delayed protection in studies conducted in vivo can be summarised as follows. Ischaemic preconditioning is capable of inducing sub-acute adaptation of myocardium which delays the death of tissue during subsequent ischaemia 24-72 hours later. This delay of tissue death is exhibited as limitation of infarct size. When the second window of protection is apparent, the extent of the protection (assessed by infarct size) is usually less than that seen following classic preconditioning. However, the duration of protection is far longer. Although the response can be observed in all species, the protection afforded against infarction may be subject to subtle but critical experimental and biological factors which may be difficult to control in all laboratories. Thus, we are dealing with a cytoprotective phenomenon which may be intrinsically weaker than classic preconditioning and which is experimentally less robust because of "masking" of protection by complex factors in the in vivo models. The use of less complex and more controllable models, such as isolated myocyte cultures, provides broad support for the existence of delayed preconditioning against ischaemic injury as observed in vivo and these studies are described below.

Table 2. Delayed preconditioning against markers of lethal ischaemic injury in vitro

Species	PC protocol	Index ischaemia	Interval	Outcome	Reference
Rat myocytes	60 min hypoxia	180 min hypoxia	24 h	Reduced CK	Yamashita [39]
Rat myocytes	20 min acidotic MI	120 min acidotic MI + NaDT	24 h	Reduced LDH More cell survival (trypan blue)	Cumming [40
Rat myocytes	2x5 min anoxia	60 min anoxia	24 h	Reduced LDH morphology ATP preservation	Zhou [41]
Rat myocytes	120 min acidotic MI	120 min acidotic MI + NaDT	24 h	Reduced CK More cell survival (MTT staining)	Heads [42]
Rat myocytes	120 min acidotic MI or 120 min hypoxia	6 h acidotic MI	24 h	Reduced CK More cell survival (MTT staining)	Heads [43]

Acidotic MI = metabolic inhibition (20 mM lactate, 10-20 mM 2-dexyglucose); NaDT = sodium dithionite 1.5 mM; CK = creatine phosphokinase; LDH = lactate dehydrogenase; MTT = methythiazoyltetrazolium

5. Delayed Preconditioning Against Myocyte Injury In Vitro

Evidence for a delayed effect of preconditioning in vitro has been obtained in isolated cardiomyocytes in several studies. Commonly, these studies screen for protection by assessing the efflux of intracellular enzymes, such as creatine phosphokinase and lactate dehydrogenase, into the culture medium. Alternative approaches are the examination of cell viability through morphological assessment (rounding of myocytes), the uptake of marker dyes, such as trypan blue, by dead or irreversibly injured cells, and the staining of viable cells by nitroblue tetrazolium (also known as MTT). Although the endpoints employed in these studies may be far removed from infarct size measured in intact tissue, they are assumed to reflect severe sarcolemmal disruption. Of course, the extent of sarcolemmal damage that predicts or constitutes irreversible cell injury is unknown. However, it is believed that a combination of two or more markers (e.g. enzyme efflux and dye penetration) will provide a reasonable index of severe ischaemic injury.

All isolated cell studies reported to date have used cardiomyocytes from neonatal tissue. Yamashita et al. [39] established that hypoxic preconditioning of rat neonatal cardiomyocytes conferred resistance to a subsequent more prolonged hypoxic period 24 hours later: there was reduced creatine phosphokinase release from myocytes preconditioned 24 hours earlier by exposure to a brief hypoxic period. Work in our laboratory examined a model of delayed protection in rat neonatal cardiomyocytes following preconditioning with 10 mM deoxyglucose and 20 mM lactate [40]. Metabolic "preconditioning" with simulated ischaemia, 24 hours before a long simulated ischaemia period, resulted in less cell death (56% cell death in preconditioned cells v 69% in non-preconditioned cells). Lactate dehydrogenase release following the "lethal" ischaemic period was also attenuated in the cells preconditioned 24 hours earlier. Zhou et al. reported that anoxic preconditioning in rat cardiomyocytes enhanced tolerance to anoxic challenge 24 hours later [41]. Most recently, Heads et al. [42, 43] have reported the use of either hypoxia or metabolic inhibition to induce delayed preconditioning in rat neonatal cardiomyocytes which is modified by selective pharmacological inhibitors of intracellular signalling pathways (see below). Together these studies in isolated cells tend to support the existence of a delayed response to preconditioning in myocardium which is able to limit the damage sustained during a subsequent hypoxic or ischaemic insult.

6. Delayed Preconditioning Against Ischaemic Injury in Other Tissues

Myocardium is not unique in exhibiting a delayed preconditioning response. There is good evidence that tissues other than myocardium may undergo sub-acute adaptation to ischaemia or hypoxia which renders them more tolerant to subsequent insult. Ischaemic preconditioning of neuronal tissue especially in the brain is well established [44]. For example, in rat brain, transient focal ischaemia resulted in greater tolerance to a subsequent ischaemic insult (Liu 1992 [45]) 72 hours later. Neuronal preconditioning shares many of the features of delayed preconditioning in myocardium in that protection is seen many hours or several days after the priming ischaemia, is associated with the induction of a cell stress response indicated by HSP70 elevation, and may even involve the activation of adenosine A_1 receptors and ATP-sensitive potassium (K_{ATP}) channel opening [46].

Ischaemia-reperfusion induces epithelial barrier dysfunction of the small intestinal mucosa. In intestinal mucosa, tolerance to ischaemia was oberved 24 hours following transient ischaemia, shown by greater resistance to ischaemia-reperfusion-induced barrier dysfunction. Interestingly this protection was observed 24 hous after preconditioning but not at one hour or 72 hours. In parallel, the antioxidant status of the mucosa was enhanced at 24 hours, but not at one hour or 72 hours after the initial ischaemic insult. Further studies indicated that the increase in antioxidant status of the mucosa observed 24 hours after the initial ischaemic insult was a result of adaptive changes in the muscular lamina propria, rather than the epithelium [47].

A report by Kume and colleagues [48] suggests that liver may also exhibit a delayed preconditioning response. Rats preconditioned with brief hepatic artery occlusion were compared with rats pretreated with heat stress or with control rats. After 48 hours recovery, rats were exposed to 30 minutes warm ischaemia and reperfusion. Both heat stress and ischaemic preconditioning attenuated the liver damage in the subsequent ischaemia-reperfusion period, improving the restoration of hepatic function during reperfusion and resulting in higher postischaemic survival. Forty eight hours after ischaemic preconditioning, HSP72 was clearly induced in the liver, as well as in the liver preconditioned with heat shock, suggesting a pattern of protection closely resembling that seen in the heart.

7. Mechanisms of Delayed Preconditioning

The last five years have seen steady progress in our understanding of the mechanisms underlying delayed preconditioning but a complete picture

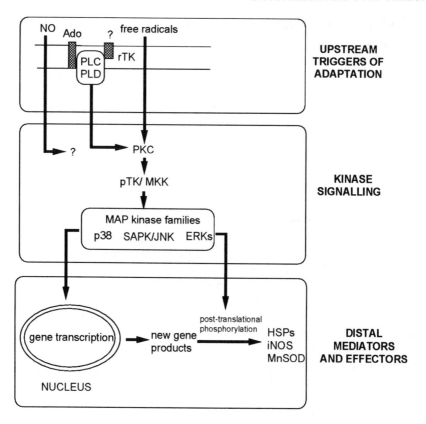

Figure 3. Schematic representation of putative mechanisms of delayed preconditioning. Upstream triggers of adaptation include adenosine (ado), nitric oxide (NO) and free radicals. It is also possible that ligands binding with receptor tyrosine kinases (rTK) may act as triggers of delayed preconditioning but there is no experimental evidence for this at present. The activation of a complex kinase signalling cascade is proposed and experimental evidence suggests the activation of protein kinase C isoforms (PKC); and tyrosine phosphorylation by protein tyrosine kinases (pTK) and MAP kinase kinases (MKK); involvement of some MAP kinase families. The identities of distal mediators and possible effectors of protection are not unequivocally established. Possible candidates include members of the heat shock protein family (HSPs), inducible nitric oxide synthase (iNOS) and manganese-dependent superoxide dismutase (Mn-SOD). The time course of protection would suggest a mechanism involving transcriptional regulation of these proteins, although it is likely that the activity of some may be regulated post-translationally.

is not yet available. The time course of delayed protection and the degree of protection afforded in the late phase, suggest that classic preconditioning and delayed preconditioning have different underlying mechanisms. However, it is clear that they do share some mechanistic features. As with classic preconditioning, mechanistic investigations have been complicated by endpoint and species considerations. Although it is likely that there may be common themes in the mechanistic pathways, it is important to qualify species and endpoint. In the following, we limit discussion of mechanisms to those studies dealing with limitation of infarction in vivo or reduction of cell death in vitro.

The paradigm that we have adopted (see figure 3) involves (i) release or activation of one or more triggers of cellular adaptation; (ii) activation of kinase cascades, acting as signalling intermediates; (iii) the upregulation of content and/or activity of distal mediators and protein effectors of protection. We will now describe current knowledge of each of these aspects.

8. Triggers of Adaptation in Delayed Preconditioning

Ischaemia-reperfusion, even when it is brief, results in a complex series of intra- and extra-cellular perturbations. Ischaemia (and subsequent reperfusion) imposes hypoxic, metabolic, osmotic and chemical stresses on the cell that result very rapidly in biochemical and biophysical changes and the generation of a number of diffusible factors. Several of these factors have been proposed to play a role in triggering delayed preconditioning against infarction and cell death. Major evidence exists for involvement of three triggering factors: adenosine, free radicals, and nitric oxide. The involvement of these three factors is described in great detail in chapters 10, 8 and 2 respectively. Here, we will summarise only the principal pieces of experimental evidence.

Adenosine

In the rabbit, adenosine release during preconditioning is an important trigger of delayed protection against infarction and this subject is covered in greater detail in chapter 10. Adenosine receptor blockade during preconditioning with the non-selective receptor antagonist 8-(p-sulphophenyl)-theophylline (SPT) abolished the protective response 24 hours later [10]. Conversely, stimulation of A_1 receptors with a selective agonist, 2-chloro-N^6-cyclopentyladenosine (CCPA), resulted in marked protection against infarction 24-72 hours later [10, 49]. Preliminary data obtained in our laboratory suggest that CCPA also induces delayed protection against infarction in the rat (see chapter 10). In the pig, delayed preconditioning *against stunning* does not appear to involve adenosine (see chapter 2) and at present it is not possible to say if this divergence is due to differences in experimental endpoint (infarction versus stunning) or species (rabbit versus pig).

Free Radicals

During oxidative stresses, such as hyperthermia or ischaemia-reperfusion, increased production of free radicals can be detected but cells may adapt biochemically by increasing the activity of the enzymes that inactivate free radicals. Thus sublethal oxidative stress may be considered to be an important trigger of adaptation. Increases in endogenous anti-oxidant protein activity, notably catalase and SOD, have been observed in many studies investigating the biology of cellular adaptation to stress. Scavenging of free radicals during preconditioning with mercaptopropionyl glycine was found to abolish the development of delayed protection against infarction in the rat, suggesting that oxidant stress during preconditioning is a trigger of delayed preconditioning in vivo [27]. Zhou et al have also presented evidence for oxidant stress involvement in delayed preconditioning against injury in anoxically preconditioned cardiomyocytes [41]. Administration of SOD during preconditioning abolished the acquisition of tolerance to anoxia 24 hours later whereas brief exposure to a superoxide generating system was able to enhance protection against anoxia 24 hours later. Of related interest, there is evidence that delayed preconditioning against tissue death in brain may also be inhibited by scavengers of free radicals [44].

Nitric Oxide

Nitric oxide is generated in ischaemic tissue and has been proposed as both a trigger and distal mediator of delayed preconditioning against infarction and stunning by Bolli's group (see chapter 2). With regard to delayed precondioning against infarction, Takano et al. have reported that L-NAME, an inhibitor of nitric oxide synthase (NOS), when administered during preconditioning abolishes delayed protection against infarction in the rabbit. Conversely, infusion of nitric oxide donors induces delayed protection [20]. Additionally, Li and Minamino [16] were able to inhibit both the development of delayed protection against infarction and the accumulation of HSP70 by administering a NOS inhibitor during preconditioning in the rabbit .

9. Signal Transduction in Delayed Preconditioning

Multiple kinase cascades are activated in response to transient ischaemia-reperfusion. The involvement of some of these kinases in the development of adaptive cardioprotection is discussed in detail in chapter 5. Below we summarise experimental evidence from our own and other laboratories for the involvement of protein kinase C (PKC), tyrosine kinases and mitogen activated protein kinase (MAP kinase) families in delayed preconditioning against infarction and cell death.

Protein Kinase C

The earliest indication that delayed preconditioning may involve PKC was obtained by Yamashita et al. [39] who showed that staurosporine, a PKC inhibitor, prevented the acquisition of delayed tolerance in hypoxically preconditioned myocytes. However the first evidence implicating a role of PKC in the mechanism of delayed protection against infarction in vivo was obtained in our rabbit model [12]. Delayed protection was abolished when preconditioning occurred in the presence of chelerythrine, a very selective PKC inhibitor. Subsequently, we observed that pretreatment of rabbits in vivo with dioctanoyl-sn-glycerol, a synthetic diacylglycerol analogue that reversibly activates PKC, resulted in an approximately 50% relative reduction in infarct size 24 hours later [50].

Direct measurements of PKC activity and translocation have not been widely studied so far but Parratt's group have recently provided evidence that sustained PKC-ε translocation to the membrane fraction occurs in the hearts of dogs subjected to rapid cardiac pacing [51], a stimulus that induces delayed protection against ischaemia-reperfusion arrhythmias. It has also been reported that brief repeated periods of coronary artery occlusion in the conscious rabbit caused the translocation of PKC-ε and η isoforms [52], and this was blocked with chelerythrine [53].

PKC could influence many nuclear transcription events either directly by phosphorylation of transcription factors, or indirectly through activation of other kinase signal cascades (e.g. Raf kinase and MAP kinase families) [54]. Certainly, there is some evidence that activation of PKC is associated with new protein synthesis or post-translational phosphorylation [55]. For example, Faucher et al. [56] have shown that a low molecular weight protein in the HSP27 family is phosphorylated by PKC in an adenocarcinoma cell line.

Other Kinase Cascades

The involvement of other parallel and downstream kinases is under investigation. Considerable interaction exists between PKC and other kinase systems including tyrosine kinases and MAP kinase cascades (see below). Tyrosine kinase activation may be an obligatory component of the signalling cascade since we observed that administration of genistein during preconditioning in rabbits abolished the delayed anti-infarct effect of preconditioning in the rabbit [13]. Additional confirmation of tyrosine phosphorylation involvement in this model has come from Kukreja's laboratory [15].

In addition to PKC and tyrosine kinases, other kinase cascades are likely to be important, especially those in MAP kinase families (see also chapter 5). Three major MAP kinase families exist in eukaryotic cells; the 'classic' p42/p44 MAP kinases (also known as p42/p44 ERKs); p38 kinase; and the stress activated c-jun N-terminal kinase (JNK, SAPK). PKC is known to phosphorylate and activate raf-1 kinase which provides a direct link to the p42/p44 MAP kinase family. There is evidence that transient ischaemia rapidly increases total MAP kinase activity in rat heart [57] (see chapter 5). Other studies in whole heart suggest the activation, by ischaemia or reactive oxygen species, of p38 kinase and JNK SAPK [58, 59] which are known to phosphorylate factors that co-ordinate gene transcription. The involvement of these kinases in delayed preconditioning is set to become the focus of increasing attention. Measurements of kinase activity and phosphorylation state are being facilitated by the availability of appropriate antibodies. Although new pharmacological tools are being introduced, the selectivity and cost of these agents may limit their use in vivo. We predict that valuable information on signalling cascades is likely to be derived from studies of delayed preconditioning in isolated cardiomyocytes. A good example of this approach has been provided recently by Heads et al. [43] who have demonstrated p38 kinase phosphorylation in isolated cardiomyocytes in response to hypoxic and metabolic preconditioning, and the abrogation of delayed protection by the p38 kinase inhibitor SB203580. Ultimately, the interactions of these complex signalling systems and their convergence on distal mediators and possible effectors of protection still needs to be evaluated.

10. Downstream Mediators and Possible Effectors of Protection

The appearance of a large number of new gene products including proto-oncogenes and regulatory proteins occurs after sublethal ischaemia as a consequence of the activation of the various signalling pathways (see chapter 6). In addition, the post-translational modification of proteins may occur, altering their biological activity. Associations between enhanced myocardial tolerance and stress-induced cytoprotective protein activity, the gradual onset of the second window of protection and the prolonged period of protection suggest that delayed preconditioning is related to changes in patterns of protein activity in the preconditioned myocardium. Almost certainly, de novo protein synthesis will be stimulated by ischaemic preconditioning but at present there is little experimental evidence from studies with transcriptional and translational inhibitors in vivo to directly support the concept that delayed preconditioning against infarction is "genomically" regulated. To date, three proteins have received most attention as possible distal mediators or effectors of delayed protection. They are: (i) members of the heat shock protein families, (ii) intracellular antioxidant enzymes, especially SOD, (iii) inducible nitric oxide synthase.

Heat Shock Proteins

As discussed in chapter 7, several lines of evidence suggest that HSP70i is a cytoprotective protein conferring tissue tolerance to ischaemia-reperfusion injury. For example, recent studies with transgenic mice that overexpress HSP70i [60-63] and studies involving transfection of the gene encoding for HSP70 into isolated myogenic cells [64, 65] and cardiomyocytes [66] show convincingly that the protein confers protection against ischaemic injury. Several reports have suggested that transient ischaemia in vivo and in isolated cells induces HSPs. Dillmann's group showed that ischaemia in canine myocardium caused increases in mRNA for HSP70 [7]. Knowlton et al. [8] reported that four 5 minute coronary occlusions followed by reperfusion in the rabbit led to an increase in HSP70i mRNA and a qualitative increase in protein immunoreactivity 24 hours later. In our group's initial report of the second window of protection [1] it was shown that elevation of HSP70i (determined by Western blot analysis) occurred in rabbit myocardium 24 hours following preconditioning. However, this particular preconditioning protocol (four 5 minute coronary occlusions) may be at the threshold for induction of HSP70i. For example, in subsequent studies with the protocol we have observed only modest HSP70i induction in rabbits preconditioned in the conscious state [18] and no induction of HSP70i in rabbits preconditioned in the anaesthetised state [67], even though the preconditoning protocol reliably confers delayed protection. It may be that subtle alterations in the protein's regulation may be relevant, such as subcellular relocalisation.

The regulation of other HSPs in response to ischaemia has been less widely investigated. HSP27 especially may be fundamental to ischaemia-induced delayed myocardial protection and protection induced by other agents. The adenosine A_1 receptor agonist, CCPA, induces delayed protection against ischaemia (see chapter 10) and although this agent does not induce HSP70i, changes in the phosphorylation state and/or translocation of HSP27, as well as induction of manganese-SOD (see below) may follow adenosine A_1 receptor activation [68].

Superoxide Dismutase

Hoshida et al. [9] described the temporal dynamics of manganese-SOD activity following preconditioning in canine myocardium and described a biphasic pattern of enzyme activity over a 24 hour period similar to the

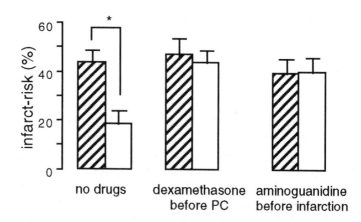

Figure 4. Pharmacological evidence implicates inducible nitric oxide synthase (NOS) in the mechanism of delayed preconditioning. Rabbits were sham operated (hatched columns) or preconditioned with four 5 minute coronary artery occlusions (open columns). Forty eight hours later, they were subjected to 30 minutes coronary occlusion. Preconditioned animals exhibited significant limitation of infarct size. Dexamethasone (4 mg/kg iv), an inhibitor of nuclear factor kappa B (NFkB) activity, given 60 minutes before preconditioning resulted in the loss of delayed protection. Aminoguanidine (300 mg/kg sc), a selective inhibitor of inducible NOS activity, 60 minutes before myocardial infarction, also resulted in loss of protection. suggests that the induction and activation of inducible NOS. Considered together the effects of these two agents suggest that the transcriptional upregulation and subsequent activation of inducible NOS may be an important mechanism in delayed preconditioning against infarction. * $P < 0.091$ vs sham.

pattern of ischaemic tolerance observed in a related study [2]. We have found that the in-gel activities of both manganese-SOD and copper-zinc-SOD are increased 24 hours after preconditioning of rabbit myocardium [67, 68]. In isolated rat cardiomyocytes, Yamashita et al. [39] reported that hypoxic preconditioning of these cells resulted in increased activity of manganese-SOD 24 hours later, at which time point marked protection was observed against a prolonged hypoxic insult. Both the rise in enzyme activity after preconditioning and the acquisition of cellular tolerance to hypoxia were abolished when myocytes were treated with staurosporine, a protein kinase inhibitor, or with anti-sense oligonucleotide directed against manganese-SOD during preconditioning.

Inducible Nitric Oxide Synthase

Nitric oxide, generated from L-arginine by nitric oxide synthases (NOSs), may under some circumstances protect against ischaemia-reperfusion. Vegh and colleagues were the first to suggest that delayed preconditioning against arrhythmias in the dog might arise as a consequence of upregulation of inducible NOS [69]. They showed that dexamethasone, an inhibitor of NOS induction, prevented the development of delayed preconditioning against arrhythmias. This important observation has been extended in both our laboratory [14] and by Bolli's group [19] (see chapter 2) to examine the possible role of inducible NOS in mediating delayed preconditioning against infarction. We found that administration of dexamethasone to rabbits before ischaemic preconditioning abolished delayed protection against infarction 48 hours later [14]. Furthermore, the administration of aminoguanidine, a selective inhibitor of inducible NOS activity, also abolished the protection (see figure 4), in general agreement with the findings of Vegh's and Bolli's groups (see chapters 2 and 4). Although questions about the specificity and selectivity of pharmacological inhibitors naturally arise, considered together the effects of these drugs support the hypothesis that the induction of inducible NOS and its subsequent activity are necessary for the development of delayed preconditioning against infarction. So far, however, there is no evidence from direct biochemical measurements that NOS activity is increased in myocardium following preconditioning at a time corresponding to protection.

11. Conclusion

Myocardium may be preconditioned by ischaemic stress in two ways: the first form of adaptation immediately confers a brief period of protection against subsequent ischaemia (classic preconditioning); the other form of adaptation confers a second window of protection against ischaemia many hours or days later. Investigation of this delayed form of preconditioning is still at an early stage. We know that during the second window of protection, myocardium shows enhanced resistance to ischaemic necrosis, ischaemia- and reperfusion-induced arrhythmias, and post-ischaemic endothelial and myocardial 'stunning'. The mechanisms of protection are not fully understood at present. There is likely to be divergence of mechanisms according to the endpoint assessed but there are undoubtedly some common features. We believe that increased resistance to ischaemia is the result of altered activity of cytoprotective proteins in the preconditioned myocardium. Some of these cytoprotective proteins may be regulated at the level of gene transcription. We hope that an understanding of the physiology and mechanisms of the second window of protection will shed light on the associations between antecedent angina pectoris and myocardial infarction (see chapter 11) and promote the rational development of new therapeutic approaches to cardioprotection based on manipulation of this innate adaptive capacity of myocardium.

Acknowledgements

The authors' work in this field during the last six years has been financially supported by a variety of agencies whom they gratefully acknowledge. Particular gratitude is due to the British Heart Foundation, the Medical Research Council of the United Kingdom, the Wellcome Trust and Glaxo-Wellcome for their generosity during this period. Dr Baxter is grateful to the British Heart Foundation for the support provided by a personal (intermediate) fellowship. The Hatter Foundation is due especial thanks for its continuing generosity. A number of current and former research students and fellows in our laboratory contributed to much of the work described here. They include Dr M S Marber, Dr R J Heads, Dr F M Goma, Dr M M Mocanu, Miss T J Pell, Dr J Imagawa and Dr A Dana. We warmly acknowledge their skill and dedication.

References

1.   Marber MS, Latchman DS, Walker JM, Yellon DM. Cardiac stress protein elevation 24 hours after brief ischemia or heat stress is associated with resistance to myocardial infarction. Circulation 1993; 88: 1264-1272.

2.   Kuzuya T, Hoshida S, Yamashita N et al. Delayed effects of sublethal ischemia on the acquisition of tolerance to ischemia. Circ Res 1993; 72: 1293-1299.

3.   Murry CE, Jennings RB, Reimer KA. Preconditioning with ischemia: a delay of lethal injury in ischemic myocardium. Circulation 1986; 74: 1124-1136.

4.   Parratt JR, Vegh A, Kaszala K, Papp JG. Protection by preconditioning and cardiac pacing against ventricular arrhythmias resulting from ischemia and reperfusion. Ann N Y Acad Sci 1996; 793: 98-107.

5.   Lawson CS, Hearse DJ. Ischemic preconditioning against arrhythmias: an anti-arrhythmic or an anti-ischemic phenomenon? Ann N Y Acad Sci 1994; 723: 138-157.

6.   Ovize M, Przyklenk K, Hale SL, Kloner RA. Preconditioning does not attenuate myocardial stunning. Circulation 1992; 85: 2247-2254.

7.   Dillmann WH, Mehta H B, Barrieux A, Guth BD, Neeley WE, Ross J. Ischemia of the dog heart induces the appearance of a cardiac mRNA coding for a protein with migration characteristics similar to the heat shock/stress protein 71. Circ Res 1986; 59: 110-114.

8.   Knowlton AA, Brecher P, Apstein CS. Rapid expression of heat shock protein in the rabbit after brief cardiac ischemia. J Clin Invest 1991; 87: 139-147.

9.   Hoshida S, Kuzuya T, Fuji H et al. Sublethal ischemia alters myocardial antioxidant activity in canine heart. Am J Physiol 1993; 264: H33-H39.

10.   Baxter GF, Marber MS, Patel VC, Yellon DM. Adenosine receptor involvement in a delayed phase of protection 24 hours following ischemic preconditioning. Circulation 1994; 90: 2993-3000.

11.   Baxter GF, Goma FM, Yellon DM. Characterisation of the infarct-limiting effect of delayed preconditioning: timecourse and dose-dependency studies in rabbit myocardium. Basic Res Cardiol 1997; 92: 159-167.

12.   Baxter GF, Goma FM, Yellon DM. Involvement of protein kinase C in the delayed cytoprotection following sublethal ischaemia in rabbit myocardium. Br J Pharmacol 1995; 115: 222-224.

13.   Imagawa J, Baxter GF, Yellon DM. Genistein, a tyrosine kinase inhibitor, blocks the "second window of protection" 48 h after ischemic preconditioning in the rabbit. J Mol Cell Cardiol 1997; 29: 1885-1893.

14.   Imagawa J, Baxter GF, Yellon DM. Delayed preconditioning against infarction may involve inducible nitric oxide synthase. Heart 1998; 79 (suppl 1): P10 (abstract).

15.   Okubo S, Bernardo NL, Jao AB, Elliott GT, Kukreja RC. Tyrosine phosphorylation is involved in second window of preconditioning in rabbit heart. Circulation 1997; 96 (suppl I): I-313 (abstract).

16.   Li W-J, Minamino T. Nitric oxide is involved in opening the second window of cardioprotection of ischemic preconditioning via induction of heat shock protein 72. Circulation 1997; 96 (suppl I): I-256 (abstract)

17.   Li W-J, Nomura Y. Nitric oxide is involved in the delayed elevation of myocardial 5'nucleotidase activity after ischemic preconditioning in rabbits. Circulation 1997; 96 (suppl I): I-256 (abstract).

18.   Yang X-M, Baxter GF, Heads RJ, Yellon DM, Downey JM, Cohen MV. Infarct limitation in the second window of protection in conscious rabbits. Cardiovasc Res 1996; 31: 777-783.

19.   Qiu Y, Rizvi A, Tang X-L et al. Nitric oxide triggers late preconditioning against myocardial infarction in conscious rabbits. Am J Physiol 1997; 273: H2931-H2936.

20.   Takano H, Manchikalapudi S, Tang X-L et al. Nitric oxide synthase is the mediator of late preconditioning against myocardial infarction in conscious rabbits. Circulation 1998; in press.

21.   Tanaka M, Fujiwara H, Yamasaki K. Ischemic preconditioning elevates cardiac stress protein but does not limit infarct size 24 or 48 h later in rabbits. Am J Physiol 1994; 267: H1476-H1482.

22.   Miki T, Swafford AN, Cohen MV, Downey JM. Second window of protection in conscious rabbits: real or artefactual. J Mol Cell Cardiol 1998; 30: A74 (abstract).

23.   Shirato C, Miura T, Ooiwa H, Toyofuku T, Wilborn WH, Downey JM. tetrazolium artifactually indicates superoxide dismutase-induced salvage in reperfused rabbit heart. J Mol Cell Cardiol 1989; 21: 1187-1193.

24.   Tanaka M, Richard VJ, Murry CE, Jennings RB, Reimer KA. Superoxide dismutase plus catalase therapy delays neither cell death nor the loss of the TTC reaction in experimental myocardial infarction in dogs. J Mol Cell Cardiol 1993; 25: 367-378.

25.   Holmbom B, Naslund U, Eriksson A, Virtanen I, Thornell L-E. Comparison of triphenyltetrazolium chloride (TTC) staining versus detection of fibronectin in experimental myocardial infarction. Histochemistry 1993; 99: 265-275.

26.   Node K, Hasegawa M, Suzuki S, Hori M. Induction of ecto-5'-nucleotidase contributes to the second-window of cardioprotection in ischemic preconditioning. Circulation 1996; 94 (suppl I): I-422 (abstract).

27.   Yamashita N, Hoshida S, Taniguchi N, Kuzuya T, Hori M. A "second window of protection" occurs 24 hours after ischemic preconditioning in rat heart. J Mol Cell Cardiol 1998; 30: in press.

28.   Kaeffer N, Richard V, Thuillez C. Delayed beneficial effects of pre-conditioning against reperfusion-induced coronary endothelial dysfunction. Evidence for a 'second window' of endothelial protection. Eur Heart J 1996; 17 (abstract suppl): 268 (abstract).

29.   Jagasia D, Whiting JM, McNulty PH. Ischemic preconditioning fails to produce a second window of protection 24 hrs later in the rat. Circulation 1996; 94 (suppl I): I-184 (abstract).

30.   Shiki K, Hearse D. Preconditioning of ischemic myocardium: reperfusion-induced arrhythmias. Am J Physiol 1987; 253: H1470-H1476.

31.   Strasser R, Arras M, Vogt A et al. Preconditioning of porcine myocardium: how much ischemia is required for induction? What is its duration? Is a renewal of effect possible? (abstract). Circulation 1994; 90 (suppl): I-109 (abstract).

32.   Qiu Y, Tang X-L, Park S-W, Sun J-Z, Kalya A, Bolli R. The early and late phases of ischemic preconditioning. A comparative analysis of their effects on infarct size, myocardial stunning, and arrhythmias in conscious pigs undergoing a 40-minute coronary occlusion. Circ Res 1997; 80: 730-742.

33.   Muller CA, Baxter GF, Latouf SE, McCarthy J, Opie LH, Yellon DM. Delayed preconditioning against infarction in pig heart after PTCA balloon inflations. J Mol Cell Cardiol 1998; 30: A74 (abstract).

34.   Kaszala K, Vegh A, Parratt JR, Papp JG. Time course of pacing-induced preconditioning in dogs. J Mol Cell Cardiol 1996; 28; 2085-2095.

35.   Sun J-Z, Tang X-L, Knowlton AA, Park S-W, Qiu Y, Bolli R. Late preconditionng against myocardial stunning: an endogenous protective mechanism that confers resistance to postischemic dysfunction 24 h after brief ischemia in conscious pigs. J Clin Invest 1995; 95: 388-403.

36.   Tang X-L, Qiu Y, Sun J-Z et al. Time-course of late preconditioning against myocardial stunning in conscious pigs. Circ Res 1996; 79: 424-434.

37.   Miura T, Adachi T, Ogawa T, Iwamoto T, Tsuchida A, Iimura O. Does myocardial stunning contribute to infarct size limitation by ischemic preconditioning? Circulation 1991; 84: 25024-2512.

38.   Hutter MM, Sievers RE, Barbosa V, Wolfe CL (1994). Heat-shock protein induction in rat hearts. A direct correlation between the amount of heat-shock protein induced and the degree of myocardial protection. Circulation 89: 355-360.

39.   Yamashita N, Nishida M, Hoshida S et al. Induction of manganese superoxide dismutase in rat cardiac myocytes increases tolerance to hypoxia 24 hours after preconditioning. J Clin Invest 1994; 94: 2193-2199.

40.   Cumming DVE, Heads RJ, Brand NJ, Yellon DM, Latchman DS. The ability of heat stress and metabolic preconditioning to protect primary rat cardiac myocytes. Basic Res Cardiol 1996; 91: 79-85.

41.   Zhou X, Zhai X, Ashraf M. Direct evidence that initial oxidtaive stress triggered by preconditioning contributes to second window of protection by endogenous antioxidant enzyme in myocytes. Circulation 1996; 93: 1177-1184.

42.   Heads RJ, Latchman DS, Marber MS. Delayed preconditioning of neonatal rat cardiocytes by simulated ischaemia: investigation of A1-receptor, alpha1-receptor and PKC involvement. Circulation 1997; 96 (suppl I): I-313 (abstract).

43.   Heads RJ, Mockridge JW, Sugden PH, Marber MS. Preconditioning of neonatal rat cardiomyocytes is associated with activation of p42/p44 MAPK and p38/RK. J Mol Cell Cardiol 1998; 30: A149 (abstract).

44.   Chen J, Simon R. Ischemic tolerance in the brain. Neurology 1997; 48: 306-311.

45.   Liu Y, Kato H, Nakata N, Kogure K. Protection of rat hippocampus against ischemic neuronal damage by pretreatment with sublethal ischemia. Brain Res 1992; 586: 121-124.

46.   Heurteaux C, Lauritzen I, Widmann C, Lazdunski M. Essential role of adenosine, adenosine A1 receptors, and ATP-sensitive K+ channels in cerebral ischemic preconditioning. Proc Natl Acad Sci USA 1995; 92: 4666-4670.

47.   Osborne DL, Aw TY, Cepinskas G, Kvietys PR. Development of ischemia-reperfusion tolerance in the rat small intestine. An epithelium-independent event. J Clin Invest 1994; 94: 1910-1918.

48.   Kume M, Yamamoto Y, Saad S et al. Ischemic preconditioning of the liver in rats: implications of heat shock protein induction to increase tolerance of ischemia-reperfusion injury. J Lab Clin Med 1996; 128: 251-258.

49.   Baxter GF, Yellon DM. Time course of delayed myocardial protection after transient adenosine A1-receptor activation in the rabbit. J Cardiovasc Pharmacol 1997; 29: 631-638.

50.   Baxter GF, Mocanu MM, Yellon DM. Attenuation of myocardial ischaemic injury 24 h after diacylglycerol treatment in vivo. J Mol Cell Cardiol 1997; 29: 1967-1975.

51.   Wilson S, Song W, Karoly K et al. Delayed cardioprotection is associated with the sub-cellular relocalisation of ventricular protein kinase C epsilon, but not p42/44MAPK. Mol Cell Biochem 1996; 160-161: 225-230.

52.   Ping P, Zhang J, Qiu Y et al. Ischemic preconditioning induces selective translocation of protein kinase C isoforms epsilon and eta in the heart of conscious rabbits without subcellular redistribution of total protein kinase C activity. Circ Res 1997; 81: 404-414.

53.   Qiu Y, Ping P, Tang X-L et al. Direct evidence that protein kinase C plays an essential role in the development of late preconditioning against myocardial stunning in conscious rabbits and that ε is the isoform involved. J Clin Invest 1998 (in press).

54.   Hug H, Sarre TF. Protein kinase C isoenzymes: divergence in signal transduction. Biochem J 1993; 291: 329-343.

55.   Issandou M, Darbon J-M. Activation of protein kinase C by phorbol esters induces DNA synthesis and protein phsophorylation in glomerular mesangial cells. FEBS Lett 1991; 281: 196-206.

56.   Faucher C, Capdevielle J, Canal I et al. The 28-kDa protein whose phosphorylation is induced by protein kinase C activatoris in MCF-7 cells belongs to the family of low molecular mass heat shock proteins and is the estrogen-regulated 24-kDa protein. J Biol Chem 1993; 268: 15168-15173.

57.   Maulik N, Watanabe M, Zu YL et al. Ischemic preconditioning triggers the activation of MAP kinases and MAPKAP kinase 2 in rat hearts. FEBS Lett 1996; 396: 233-237.

58.   Knight RJ, Buxton DB. Stimulation of c-Jun kinase and mitogen-activated protein kinase by ischemia and reperfusion in the perfused rat heart. Biochem Biophys Res Commun 1996; 218: 83-88.

59.   Bogoyevitch MA, Gillespie-Brown J, Ketterman AJ et al. Stimulation of the stress-activated mitogen-activated protein kinase subfamilies in perfused heart. p38/RK mitogen-activated protein kinases and c-Jun N-terminal kinases are activated by ischemia/reperfusion. Circ Res 1996; 79: 162-173.

60.   Marber MS, Mestril R, Chi S-H, Sayen R, Yellon DM, Dillmann WH. Over-expression of the rat inducible 70-kD heat stress protein in a transgenic mouse increases the resistance of the heart to ischemic injury. J Clin Invest 1995; 95: 1446-1456.

61.   Plumier J-CL, Ross BM, Currie RW et al. Transgenic mice exprssing the human heat shock protein 70 have improved post-ischemic myocardial recovery. J Clin Invest 1995; 95: 1854-1860.

62.   Radford NB, Fina M, Benjamin IJ et al.Cardioprotective effects of 70-kDa heat shock protein in transgenic mice. Proc Natl Acad Sci USA 1996; 93: 2339-2342.

63.   Hutter JJ, Mestril R, Tam EK, Sievers RE, Dillmann WH, Wolfe CL. Overexpression of heat shock protein 72 in transgenic mice decreases infarct size in vivo. Circulation1996; 94: 1408-1411.

64.   Mestril R, Chi S-H, Sayen M R, O'Reilly K, Dillmann W H. Expression of inducible stress protein 70 in rat heart myogenic cells confers protection against simulated ischemia induced injury. J Clin Invest 1994; 93: 759-767.

65.   Heads RJ, Yellon DM, Latchman DS. Differentinal cytoprotection against heat stress or hypoxia following expression of specific stress protein genes in myogenic cells. J Mol Cell Cardiol 1995; 27: 1669-1678.

66.   Cumming DVE, Heads RJ, Watson A, Latchman DS, Yellon DM. Differential protection of primary rat cardiocytes by transfection of specific heat stress proteins. J Mol Cell Cardiol 1996; 27:

67.   Heads RJ, Baxter GF, Yellon DM. Changes in the activity of SOD and subcellular distribution of HSP70 and HSP27 during delayed ischaemic preconditioning in rabbit heart. J Mol Cell Cardiol 1996; 28: A31 (abstract).

68.   Heads RJ, Baxter GF, Latchman DS, Yellon DM. Delayed protection in rabbit heart following ischaemic preconditioning is associated with modulation of HSP27 and superoxide dismutase at 24 hours. J Mol Cell Cardiol 1995; 27: A163 (abstract).

69.   Vegh A, Papp JG, Parratt JR. Prevention by dexamethasone of the marked antiarrhythmic effects of preconditioning induced 20 h after rapid cardiac pacing. Br J Pharmacol 1994; 113: 1081-1082.

2

Delayed Preconditioning Against Myocardial Stunning: Role of Nitric Oxide as Trigger and Mediator

R Bolli, B Dawn, X-L Tang, Y Qiu, P Ping, J Zhang and H Takano

1. Introduction

Ischaemic preconditioning (PC) induces two temporally-distinct phases of cardioprotection: an early phase, which develops within minutes from the initial ischemic insult and lasts 2-3 hours, and a late (or delayed) phase, which becomes apparent 12-24 hours later and lasts for 3-4 days (reviewed in references 1 and 2). These two phases have different pathophysiology and probably different mechanisms. Since the late phase lasts much longer, it may have greater clinical relevance [1,2]. The late phase of ischaemic PC has been found to protect not only against myocardial infarction, but also against reversible postischaemic myocardial dysfunction (myocardial stunning) [1,2]. The purpose of this chapter is to succinctly review the existing knowledge regarding the pathophysiology and pathogenesis of late PC against myocardial stunning and to summarise recent evidence supporting a major role of nitric oxide (NO) in the late phase of ischaemic PC ("nitric oxide hypothesis of late PC").

2. Pathophysiology of Late Preconditioning Against Stunning

Description of the Phenomenon

Although the early phase of ischaemic PC provides powerful protection against infarction, it has generally been found to be ineffective in protecting against myocardial stunning [1, 2]. We hypothesised that a sublethal ischaemic insult may induce cellular adaptations that protect against the development of stunning after subsequent exposure to ischaemia, but that these adaptations develop slowly and require several hours to become manifest. We initially tested this hypothesis in conscious pigs subjected to a sequence of ten 2 minute coronary occlusions interspersed with 2 minute reperfusion intervals [3]. We found that this sequence induced severe myocardial stunning, but when the same sequence was repeated 24 hours later, the severity of stunning was markedly reduced (by approximately 50%) (Figure 1). This protection dissipated within ten days after the last ischaemic stress, but could be reinduced by another sequence of ten 2 minute occlusion/2 minute reperfusion cycles. To determine whether late PC against stunning was dependent upon unique characteristics of the pig, we investigated this phenomenon in conscious rabbits subjected to a sequence of six 4 minute coronary occlusions/4 minute reperfusion cycles for three consecutive days (day 1, 2, and 3) [4]. Again, we found that the severity of myocardial stunning induced by the sequence of ischaemic episodes was decreased by approximately 50% on days 2 and 3 compared with day 1 [4]. Thus, the same phenomenon initially observed in pigs was also observed in rabbits. The fact that late PC against stunning occurs in two different species (pigs and rabbits) suggests that it is species-independent. The reproducibility of late PC against stunning is noteworthy; in both the pig and the rabbit studies, we have consistently observed this phenomenon in every animal studied thus far.

Time Course

A series of studies was performed to assess the time course of late PC against stunning [4,5]. In conscious pigs, we found that the protection was not yet present at 6 hours after the last ischaemic episode, became partially manifest at 12 hours, achieved full expression at 24 hours, lasted for at least 3 days, and disappeared within 6 days from the PC ischaemia [5]. We have subsequently observed a similar time course in conscious rabbits. Specifically, late PC was still present 72 hours after the initial ischaemic stimulus but was no longer present at 96 hours [4].

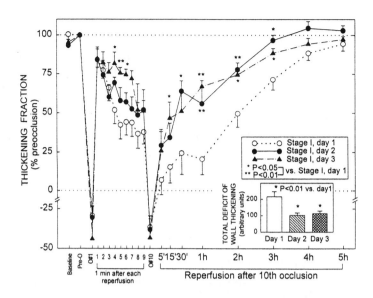

Figure 1. Systolic thickening fraction in the ischaemic-reperfused region of conscious pigs subjected to a sequence of ten 2 minute coronary occlusion/2 minute reperfusion cycles. Shown are the measurements of thickening fraction obtained at baseline, immediately before the 1st occlusion (pre-occlusion, pre-O), 1 minute into the 1st coronary occlusion (O#1), 1 minute into each of the first nine reperfusions, 1 minute into the 10th occlusion (O#10), and at selected times during the 5 hour reperfusion interval following the 10th coronary occlusion: open circles indicate measurements taken on day 1; closed circles, measurements taken on day 2; and closed triangles, measurements taken on day 3. Thickening fraction is expressed as a percentage of preocclusion values. **Inset.** Total deficit of wall thickening during the 5 hour reperfusion period following the 10th reperfusion. The total deficit of wall thickening is an integrated measure of the overall severity of myocardial stunning. Total deficits were similar and significantly less on day 2 and day 3 compared to day 1, demonstrating the protective effect of late PC against stunning. Data are means ± SEM. Note that the recovery of thickening fraction was markedly enhanced on days 2 and 3 compared with day 1, indicating the development of a late PC effect against myocardial stunning. (Reproduced from Sun et al, J Clin Invest 1995; 95: 388-403, by copyright permission of the Rockefeller University Press).

Dose-Related or All-or-None Phenomenon?

In our initial studies in conscious rabbits [4], we found that when the sequence of six 4 minute coronary occlusion/4 minute reperfusion cycles was repeated for four consecutive days, the magnitude of the PC effect did not increase from the second to the fourth day, suggesting that the protection observed on the second day is maximal or near maximal. We have subsequently obtained evidence that late PC against stunning is an all-or-none phenomenon [6]. Specifically, we found in conscious rabbits that one or two   4 minute coronary occlusion/4 minute reperfusion cycles on day 1 were not sufficient to induce any PC effect on day 2. A clear-cut protection developed when the rabbits were subjected to three 4 minute occlusion/4 minute reperfusion cycles on day 1. However, the magnitude of this protection could not be increased by preconditioning the rabbits with six or even twelve 4 minute occlusion/4 minute reperfusion cycles on day 1 [6]. Thus, a sharp threshold exists for the induction of late PC against stunning: as the number of occlusion/reperfusion cycles increases from two to three, there is an abrupt transition from no protection to full protection.

We now turn to discuss the mechanism of late preconditioning against stunning. Despite intense research, the mechanism of the late phase of ischaemic PC remains elusive [1, 2]. For the sake of clarity, it is useful to subdivide this mechanism into three distinct components: the triggering events, the signal transduction pathways, and the mediation of protection.

3. The Preconditioning Stimulus or 'Trigger' of Late PC

A number of chemical signals have been proposed to trigger the development of the late phase of ischaemic PC.

Adenosine

It is well established that stimulation of adenosine A_1 receptors can initiate early PC [7]. Baxter et al,[8] have shown that activation of adenosine A_1 receptors can also initiate late PC against infarction in rabbits. However, we have found that blockade of adenosine receptors with two different non-selective antagonists 8-(p-sulfophenyl)-theophylline (SPT) and PD 115,199 (both of which block A_1, A_2, and A_3 receptors), failed to prevent the development of late PC against myocardial stunning in conscious rabbits, and that activation of adenosine A_1 receptors with 2-chloro-N^6-cyclopentyladenosine (CCPA) failed to induce late PC against stunning [9]. Thus, adenosine receptors are not involved in the development of late PC against stunning in conscious rabbits.

Reactive Oxygen Species

Although the generation of reactive oxygen species (ROS) after ischaemia-reperfusion has generally been viewed as a deleterious

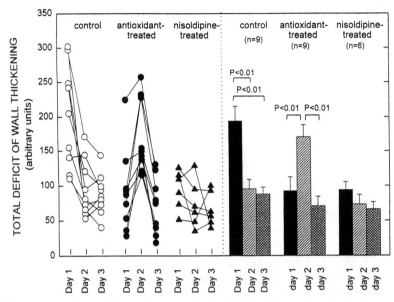

Figure 2. Total deficit of systolic wall thickening in conscious pigs subjected to a sequence of ten 2 minute coronary occlusion/2 minute reperfusion cycles on days 1, 2 and 3 in the control, antioxidant-treated, and nisoldipine-treated groups. The values of total deficit of wall thickening in individual pigs are illustrated in the left panel; the mean (± SEM) values of total deficit of wall thickening in each group are depicted in the right panel. In contrast to control pigs, in which the recovery of wall thickening was enhanced on day 2 compared with day 1, in antioxidant-treated pigs the recovery of wall thickening was enhanced on day 1 and significantly worse on day 2, indicating that administration of antioxidants had a protective effect against myocardial stunning on day 1, but abrogated the development of late PC on day 2 (the results in the control group were similar to those illustrated in Figure 1). (Reproduced from Sun et al, J Clin Invest 1996; 97: 562-576, by copyright permission of the Rockefeller University Press).

phenomenon, mounting evidence indicates that ROS can also serve as important intracellular signalling molecules. We have found in conscious pigs that administration of antioxidant therapy, namely superoxide dismutase (SOD) plus catalase plus mercapto-propionylglycine (MPG), during the initial ischaemic challenge on day 1 completely prevents the development of late PC against myocardial stunning on day 2 (Figure 2) [10], indicating that the generation of ROS during the PC ischaemia plays an essential role in triggering this cardioprotective response. In subsequent studies in conscious rabbits, we have found that the development of late PC against stunning is blocked by MPG alone, but not by SOD alone or catalase alone, implicating MPG-sensitive oxidants (hydroxyl radical [·OH] and/or peroxynitrite [ONOO⁻]) in the initiation of late PC [11]. In the absence of ischaemia, intracoronary administration of an ROS-generating solution in rabbits induces a late PC effect against stunning that is indistinguishable from that observed after ischemic PC [12]. Taken together, these data indicate an important role of ROS in triggering late PC against stunning.

Nitric Oxide

Approximately 2 years ago, we postulated that one possible source of the ROS that trigger late PC is NO. NO is produced by the oxidation of L-arginine by a family of nitric oxide synthase (NOS) isoenzymes that includes two constitutive isoforms, namely endothelial NOS (eNOS) and neuronal (or brain) NOS (bNOS), and an inducible isoform (iNOS) [13,14]. eNOS, which is expressed not only in endothelial cells, but also in cardiac myocytes, produces NO via a complex reaction that is stimulated by calcium and requires NADPH, among other co-factors [13]. Reperfusion following transient ischaemia could stimulate rapid NO synthesis by providing the oxygen needed to produce NO, since calcium and NADPH have already been made available by the ischaemic insult. At the same time, production of superoxide anion ($\cdot O_2^-$) is also accelerated in the early phase of reperfusion [15]. $\cdot O_2^-$ and NO react rapidly to form ONOO$^-$, which then protonates and decomposes to generate $\cdot$OH or some other potent oxidant with similar reactivity [16]. $\cdot$OH or other NO-derived oxidants could then trigger late PC.

On the basis of these considerations, we hypothesised that generation of NO during the first ischaemic stress triggers the development of late PC against myocardial stunning 24 hours later [17]. To test this hypothesis, we administered N^ω-nitro-L-arginine (L-NA), a non-selective inhibitor of all three NOS isoforms, in conscious rabbits undergoing a sequence of six 4 minute occlusion/4 minute reperfusion cycles on three consecutive days [17]. We found that administration of L-NA on day 1 completely blocked the development of late PC against myocardial stunning on day 2 (Figure 3), demonstrating that this cardioprotective phenomenon is triggered by NO generated during the initial PC ischaemia. We have subsequently found that administration of L-NA before the PC ischaemia also blocked the development of late PC against myocardial infarction 24 hours later in conscious rabbits [18]. The concept that NO serves as the trigger of late PC is further supported by our observation that pretreatment with two structurally-unrelated NO donors, diethylenetriamine/NO (DETA-NO) and S-nitroso-N-penicillamine (SNAP), induces a delayed protective effect against both myocardial stunning and infarction that is indistinguishable from that observed during the late phase of ischaemic PC. Therefore, the generation of NO during the PC ischaemia serves as the trigger not only for late PC against stunning, but also for late PC against infarction, indicating that

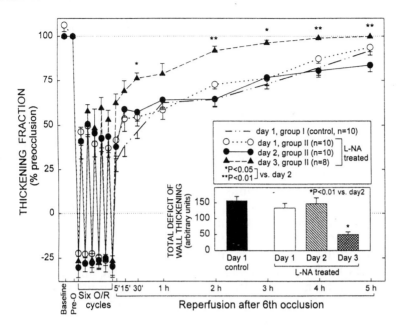

Figure 3. Systolic thickening fraction in the ischaemic-reperfused region in L-NA treated rabbits before administration of L-NA (baseline), 9 minutes after the end of the infusion of L-NA (immediately before the first occlusion) (preocclusion [Pre-O]), 3 minutes into each coronary occlusion (O), 3 minutes into each reperfusion (R), and at selected times during the 5 hour reperfusion interval following the sixth occlusion. Open circles indicate measurements taken on day 1; closed circles, measurements taken on day 2; and closed triangles, measurements taken on day 3. To facilitate comparisons, the data pertaining to day 1 of the control group are also shown (thick interrupted line without symbols). Thickening fraction is expressed as a percentage of Pre-O values. Data are mean ± SEM. In contrast to control rabbits, in which the recovery of wall thickening was markedly enhanced on day 2 compared with day 1, in L-NA-treated rabbits, the recovery of wall thickening was similar on days 1 and 2, indicating that L-NA abrogated the development of late PC against stunning. **Inset.** Total deficit of wall thickening during the 5 hour reperfusion period following the 6th reperfusion. The total deficit of wall thickening is an integrated measure of the overall severity of myocardial stunning. Notice that the total deficits were similar on day 1 and day 2, indicating that L-NA prevented late PC against stunning. (Reproduced with permission of the American Heart Association from Bolli et al, Circ Res 1997; 81: 42-52).

this radical plays a key role in the delayed myocardial adaptation to ischaemic stress.

The source of increased NO formation during the PC ischaemia is likely to be the constitutively-expressed eNOS, which has been identified both in endothelial cells and in cardiac myocytes [13, 14]. This concept is supported by our finding that the development of late PC against stunning in conscious rabbits was blocked by the non-selective NOS antagonist L-

NA, but not by the relatively-selective iNOS antagonists aminoguanidine and S-methylisothiourea [17,40]. Ischaemic PC could stimulate constitutively-expressed eNOS by at least three mechanisms: (i) ischaemia-induced increases in intracellular calcium and NADPH; (ii) increased shear stress during the repeated reactive hyperaemias and/or; (iii) release of bradykinin with activation of endothelial B_2 receptors [19]. We propose that generation of NO results in a signalling cascade that culminates in increased gene transcription and synthesis of cardioprotective protein(s). Several transcription factors, enzymes, receptors, G proteins, protein kinases, protein phosphatases, and ion channels are known to be modulated by NO [13,14]. NO could also modulate gene expression through the formation of ONOO- and/or secondary ROS, which in turn could act via activation of protein kinase C [20] or a cis-acting regulatory element (antioxidant responsive element) that mediates cellular responses to oxidative stress [21]. Further studies will be necessary to elucidate the mechanism whereby NO induces late PC against both stunning and infarction, and also to determine whether this phenomenon is triggered by NO itself or by one of its byproducts (such as ONOO-).

In summary, in the conscious rabbit, NO (presumably generated by eNOS) is the trigger that initiates the development of late PC both against myocardial stunning and against myocardial infarction.

4. The Signal Transduction Pathways of Late PC

It is now clear that brief PC episodes of ischaemia activate a complex intracellular signalling cascade. While the exact nature of the signal transduction pathways underlying the development of late PC remain unclear at this time, several kinase systems are likely to be involved.

Protein Kinase C

Protein kinase C (PKC) has been proposed as one of the key elements involved in signal transduction in both the early and the late phase of ischaemic PC [7, 22-24]. The evidence supporting a role of PKC in ischaemic PC, however, is indirect, being based on pharmacological studies in which the PC protection was abrogated by PKC antagonists and, conversely, the PC effect was mimicked by PKC activators [7, 22-24]. Furthermore, the PKC hypothesis, particularly in relation to early PC, is controversial since it is supported by some studies [7, 22] but not by others [25, 26]. To directly test the PKC hypothesis of ischaemic PC, we performed a series of studies in which the expression and subcellular distribution of all eleven PKC isoforms were systematically analysed in conscious rabbits subjected to ischaemic PC in the presence and absence of PKC inhibitors. We found that ischaemic PC induces isoform-selective translocation of the ε and η isozymes of PKC without changes in total myocardial PKC activity or in its subcellular distribution, indicating that activation of PKC by ischaemic PC is isoform-selective and that measurements of total PKC activity are not sufficiently sensitive to detect the involvement of PKC in PC [27]. We subsequently demonstrated that chelerythrine (a specific PKC inhibitor), at a dose that blocks the translocation of both PKC ε and η (5 mg/kg), also blocks the development of late PC against myocardial stunning [24, 28]. In contrast, a ten-fold lower dose (0.5 mg/kg), which blocks the translocation of PKC η but not that of PKC ε, failed to block late PC against myocardial stunning, indicating that the translocation of PKC ε is necessary for late PC to occur whereas that of PKC η is not [28]. Taken together, these results [27,28] indicate that PKC plays an essential role in the late phase of ischaemic PC and specifically implicate one novel isoform (the ε isoform) in the development of this phenomenon.

Downstream Kinases

The downstream targets of PKC phosphorylation remain unknown. We have recently demonstrated that ischaemic PC activates the p44/p42 mitogen-activated protein kinases (MAPKs), the p46/p54 JNKs, and possibly the p38 MAPK [29, 30], and that selective overexpression of PKC ε in isolated cardiac myocytes induces a marked activation of p44/p42 MAPKs and p46/p54 JNKs [31]. These findings are compatible with the hypothesis that PKC-dependent signalling in ischaemic PC may involve the MAPK family of enzymes, but further studies using MAPK inhibitors will be necessary to elucidate this issue.

5. The Mediator(s) of the Protective Effects of Late PC

Perhaps the most important unresolved issue pertaining to late PC is the identity of the mediator(s) that confers resistance to myocardial ischaemia 24 hours after the initial PC stimulus. The fact that the protective effect requires 12-24 hours to develop and lasts for 3-4 days is consistent with the synthesis and degradation of cardioprotective protein(s). We have recently demonstrated that the same protocol that triggers late PC against stunning and infarction (six 4 minute occlusion/4 minute reperfusion cycles) causes a rapid, marked increase in the rate of myocardial protein synthesis, and that blocking such an increase with cycloheximide blocks the development of late PC [32]. Thus, late PC requires increased synthesis of new proteins, not simply activation of pre-existing proteins. The nature of the protein(s) synthesised in response to ischaemic PC remains unclear. Several hypotheses have been proposed.

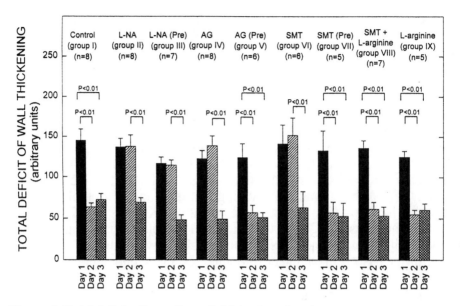

Figure 4. Total deficit of systolic wall thickening after the sixth reperfusion on days 1, 2 and 3 in nine groups of rabbits. Rabbits in group I received no treatment. Rabbits in groups II (L-NA), IV (AG), and VI (SMT) received intravenous dose(s) of L-NA, AG, and SMT, respectively, 10 minutes before the first coronary occlusion on day 2. Rabbits in groups III (L-NA-pre), V (AG-pre), and VII (SMT-pre) received similar intravenous doses of L-NA, AG, and SMT, respectively, 10 minutes before the first coronary occlusion on day 1. Rabbits in group VIII received an intravenous infusion of L-arginine starting 28 minutes before the first coronary occlusion SMT + L-arginine-treated, and L-arginine-treated groups (groups I, II, III, IV, V, VI, VII, VIII and IX, respectively) of rabbits. Data are mean ± SEM. Pre indicates pretreatment. Administration of either a nonselective (L-NA) or an iNOS-selective (AG and SMT) NOS inhibitor on day 2 completely abrogated late PC against myocardial stunning (groups II, IV, and VI, respectively), indicating that NOS (probably iNOS) is the mediator of this cardioprotective phenomenon. The abrogation of late PC by SMT was completely reversed by L-arginine (group VIII), indicating that SMT acted specifically by inhibiting NOS activity. (Reproduced with permission of the American Heart Association from Bolli et al., Circ Res 1997; 81: 1094-1107).

Heat Shock Proteins

A family of proteins known as the heat shock proteins (HSPs) has been shown to be expressed in the heart exposed to non-lethal heat stress [33]. Several studies have demonstrated that ischaemic PC protocols induce upregulation of HSPs in the heart after 24 hours or longer, concomitant with the development of a protective effect (reviewed in reference 33). Direct evidence for a cardioprotective role of HSPs has been provided by studies in transgenic mice overexpressing HSP70, in

which the heart was found to be relatively resistant to
ischaemia/reperfusion injuries in various settings [34]. The critical,
unresolved issue is whether blocking upregulation of HSPs following
ischaemic PC results in abrogation of late PC.

Antioxidants

Since ROS (which are generated during the ischaemic PC stimulus) can
upregulate antioxidant enzymes, and since ROS play a major causative
role in myocardial stunning [35, 36], it seemed logical to postulate that the
protective effects of late PC are mediated by increased activity of one or
more antioxidant enzymes. This hypothesis was further supported by the
finding of increased myocardial activity of Mn SOD 24 hours after PC in
dogs [37] and of Mn SOD and Cu-Zn SOD 24 hours after ischaemic PC
in rabbits [38]. However, to our surprise (and disappointment), we found
in conscious pigs that there was no increase in Mn SOD, Cu-Zn SOD,
catalase, glutathione peroxidase, or glutathione reductase 24 hours after
ischaemic PC [39]. We have recently obtained similar findings in
conscious rabbits. Therefore, late PC against myocardial stunning is not
mediated by increased endogenous antioxidant defences.

Nitric Oxide

NO, or its second messenger cGMP, has been shown to exert a number
of actions that would be expected to be beneficial during myocardial
ischaemia, including antagonism of the effects of beta-adrenergic
stimulation, inhibition of calcium influx into myocytes, decrease in
myocardial contractility, and reduction in myocardial oxygen consumption
[13,14]. Accordingly, we hypothesised that the protective effects of late
PC are mediated by augmented NO formation secondary to ischaemia-
induced alterations of NOS gene expression. We tested this hypothesis
indirectly using a pharmacological approach. We examined the effects on
late PC of NOS antagonists administered on day 2 (i.e. after the PC effect
has already been triggered by the first ischaemic challenge but prior to the
second ischaemic challenge). Administration of the non-selective NOS
inhibitor L-NA completely abrogated late PC against stunning in
conscious rabbits (Figure 4) [40], indicating that the protection afforded
by late PC is a NOS-dependent phenomenon. Administration of the
relatively-selective iNOS inhibitors aminoguanidine (AG) and S-
methylisothiourea on day 2 also abrogated late PC against myocardial
stunning (Figure 4) [40], indicating that the specific isoform involved
in mediating the protective effects of late PC is iNOS. In a more recent
study [41], administration of either AG or L-NA prior to a 30 minute
coronary occlusion on day 2 completely blocked the protective effects of
late PC against infarction in conscious rabbits, indicating that the activity

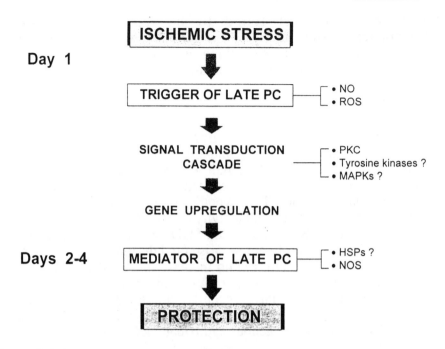

Figure 5. Schematic representation of the pathways involved in the genesis of late preconditioning against myocardial stunning. A brief episode of myocardial ischaemia/reperfusion causes increased production of NO and reactive oxygen species (ROS), which serve as triggers for the development of late PC. NO and ROS activate a complex signal transduction cascade (which involves PKC, tyrosine kinases, and possibly MAPKs), which leads to activation of transcription factors, upregulation of cardioprotective genes, and increased activity of NOS 24-72 hours later. This increased NOS activity confers protection during the second ischaemic stress.

of NOS is necessary to mediate not only the attenuation of myocardial stunning, but also the infarct-sparing effects of late PC. None of the NOS inhibitors had any appreciable effect on either myocardial stunning or myocardial infarction in nonpreconditioned hearts [40,41]. Taken together, these results indicate that the cardioprotective effects of late PC are mediated by the activity of NOS and, specifically, iNOS. In conclusion, NO plays a dual role in the pathophysiology of the late phase of ischaemic PC, acting initially as the trigger and subsequently as the mediator of the protection.

6. The Nitric Oxide Hypothesis of Late PC

A summary of our current understanding of the pathophysiology of the late phase of ischaemic PC is illustrated in Figures 5 and 6. We propose

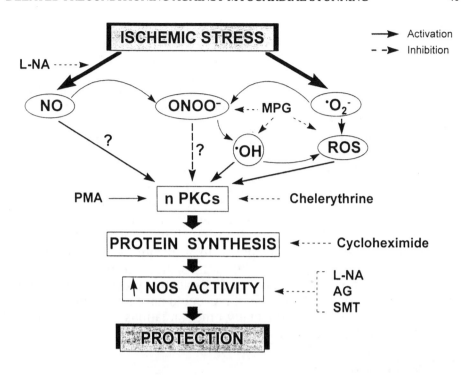

Figure 6. Schematic representation of the cellular mechanisms involved in triggering late PC against myocardial stunning. A brief episode of myocardial ischaemia/reperfusion causes increased production of NO and $\cdot O_2^-$, which then react to form $\cdot ONOO^-$. $\cdot ONOO^-$, in turn, activates the novel subgroup of PKCs (most likely PKC ε) either directly or via its reactive byproducts, such as $\cdot OH$. $\cdot O_2^-$ could also generate secondary ROS capable of activating nPKCs. PKC activation results in increased synthesis of new proteins and increased NOS activity on day 2, which is responsible for the protection. According to this paradigm, late PC against stunning can be abrogated by blocking increased NO synthesis following the initial stress with L-NA on day 1, by scavenging reactive species derived from NO (MPG on day 1), by inhibiting nPKCs (chelerythrine on day 1), by inhibiting protein synthesis (cycloheximide on day 1), or by blocking the enhanced NOS activity on day 2 (L-NA, AG, or SMT on day 2). Conversely, administration of PMA on day 1 can bypass the triggering events and activate the development of late PC in the absence of ischaemia.

that a brief ischaemic stress causes a burst of NO production (probably via eNOS) as well as $\cdot O_2^-$ production. NO and $\cdot O_2^-$ could then react to form $ONOO^-$, which could then activate PKC, either directly or via secondary byproducts such as $\cdot OH$. Both NO and ROS could also stimulate PKC independently. Activation of PKC triggers a complex signal transduction cascade which leads to transcriptional activation of the iNOS gene, increased iNOS protein and activity, and increased generation of NO during the second ischaemic challenge. According to this paradigm, NO plays two completely different roles in late PC: on day 1, it initiates the development of the cardioprotective mechanism, whereas on day 2, it protects against myocardial stunning. We propose that two different NOS isoforms are sequentially involved in the pathophysiological cascade of late PC, with eNOS generating the NO that initiates the development of the PC response on day 1 and iNOS then generating the NO that protects against recurrent ischaemia on day 2. Previous studies have documented that NO exerts a variety of biological actions resulting in rapid but transient physiological responses [13,14]. The results summarised in this chapter support a novel pathophysiological paradigm in which NO acts as an intracellular signal that modulates cardiac gene expression in response to ischaemia and possibly other stresses, resulting in delayed but long-lasting cellular adaptations mediated by de novo synthesis of cardioprotective protein(s). This novel, previously unrecognised function of NO could have implications not only for ischaemic PC but also for many other situations that are associated with enhanced NOS activity.

7. Conclusions

The late phase of ischaemic PC against myocardial stunning is a long-lasting (at least 72 hours), powerful (approximately 50% reduction in total dysfunction), and highly reproducible cardioprotective mechanism that has been observed in two different animal species (pigs and rabbits). While the exact cellular and molecular mechanisms underlying this phenomenon remain to be deciphered, it is clear that NO plays a prominent role both in initiating and in mediating this cardioprotective response. Accordingly, late PC against myocardial stunning can be viewed as a NO-dependent phenomenon. Unravelling the cellular mechanisms responsible for late PC against myocardial stunning will not only enhance our understanding of the manner in which brief ischaemic stresses affect cardiac gene expression, but may also have therapeutic implications for the development of pharmacological strategies capable of mimicking the beneficial effects of late PC.

Acknowledgements

We gratefully acknowledge Trudy Keith for expert secretarial assistance. This work was supported in part by NIH ROl grants HL-43151 and HL-55757 (Dr. Bolli) and R29 HL-58166 (Dr. Ping), by National AHA

Award 9750721N (Dr. Ping), and by the Medical Research Grant Program of the Jewish Hospital Foundation, Louisville, KY.

References

1.   Bolli R. The early and late phases of preconditioning against myocardial stunning and the essential role of oxyradicals in the late phase: an overview. Basic Res Cardiol 1996; 91: 57-63.

2.   Bolli R, Tang X-L, Qiu Y, Park S-W. The late phase of preconditioning against myocardial stunning. In Mentzer RM, Kitakaze M, Downey JM, Hori M (editors): Adenosine, cardioprotection and its clinical application. Kluwer Academic Publishers, Boston, 1997, 29-35.

3.   Sun J-Z, Tang X-L, Knowlton AA, Park S-W, Qiu Y, Bolli R. Late preconditioning against myocardial stunning: An endogenous protective mechanism that confers resistance to postischemic dysfunction 24 hours after brief ischemia in conscious pigs. J Clin Invest 1995; 95: 388-403.

4.   Qiu Y, Maldonado C, Tang X-L, Bolli R. Late preconditioning against myocardial stunning in conscious rabbits. Circulation 1995; 93 (Suppl I): I-388 (abstract).

5.   Tang X-L, Qiu Y, Park SW, Sun J-Z, Kalya A, Bolli R. Time-course of late preconditioning against myocardial stunning in conscious pigs. Circ Res 1996; 79: 424-434.

6.   Teschner S, Qiu Y, Tang X-L et al. Late preconditioning against myocardial stunning in conscious rabbits: a dose-related or all-or-none phenomenon? Circulation 1996; 94 (Suppl I): I-423 (abstract).

7.   Downey JM, Cohen MV, Ytrehus K, Liu Y. Cellular mechanisms in ischemic preconditioning: The role of adenosine and protein kinase C. Ann N Y Acad Sci 1994; 723: 82-98.

8.   Baxter GF, Marber MS, Patel VC, Yellon DM. Adenosine receptor involvement in a delayed phase of myocardial protection 24 hours after ischemic preconditioning. Circulation 1994; 90: 2993-3000.

9.   Maldonado C, Qiu Y, Tang X-L, Cohen MV, Auchampach J, Bolli R. Role of adenosine receptors in late preconditioning against myocardial stunning in conscious rabbits. Am J Physiol 1997; 273: H1324-H1332.

10.   Sun J-Z, Tang X-L, Park SW, Qiu Y, Turrens JF, Bolli R. Evidence for an essential role of reactive oxygen species in the genesis of late preconditioning against myocardial stunning in conscious pigs. J Clin Invest 1996; 97: 562-576.

44

R. BOLLI ET AL.

11.   Tang X-L, Rizvi AN, Qiu Y et al. Evidence that the hydroxyl radical triggers late preconditioning against myocardial stunning in conscious rabbits. Circulation 1997; 96 (Suppl I): I-255 (abstract).

12.   Takano H, Tang X-L, Qiu Y et al. Intracoronary administration of oxygen radicals induces late preconditioning against stunning in conscious rabbits. Circulation 1997; 96 (Suppl I): I-256-57 (abstract).

13.   Gross SS, Wolin MS. Nitric oxide: Pathophysiological mechanisms. Annu Rev Physiol 1995; 57: 737-769.

14.   Kelly RA, Balligand JL, Smith TW. Nitric oxide and cardiac function. Circ Res 1996; 79: 363-380.

15.   Zweier JL, Broderick R, Kuppusamy P, Thompson-Gorman S, Lutty GA, Determination of the mechanism of free radical generation in human aortic endothelial cells exposed to anoxia and reoxygenation. J Biol Chem 1994; 269: 24156-24162.

16.   Beckman JS, Beckman TW, Chen J, Marshall PA, Freeman BA. Apparent hydroxyl radical production by peroxynitrite: implications for endothelial injury from nitric oxide and superoxide. Proc Natl Acad Sci U.S.A. 1990; 87: 1620-1624.

17.   Bolli R, Bhatti ZA, Tang X-L et al. Evidence that late preconditioning against myocardial stunning in conscious rabbits is triggered by the generation of nitric oxide. Circ Res 1997; 81: 42-52.

18.   Qiu Y, Rizvi A, Tang X-L et al. Nitric oxide triggers late preconditioning against myocardial infarction in conscious rabbits. Am J Physiol 1997; 273: H2931-H2936.

19.   Moncada S, Higgs A. The L-arginine-nitric oxide pathway. N Engl J Med 1993; 329: 2002-2012.

20.   Gopalakrishna R, Anderson WB. Ca^{2+}- and phospholipid-independent activation of protein kinase C by selective oxidative modification of the regulatory domain. Proc Natl Acad Sci USA 1989; 86: 6758-6762.

21.   Rushmore TH, Morton MR, Pickett CB. The antioxidant responsive element: activation by oxidative stress and identification of the DNA consensus sequence required for functional activity. J Biol Chem 1991; 266: 11632-11639.

22.   Ytrehus Y, Liu Y, Downey JM. Preconditioning protects ischemic rabbit heart by protein kinase C activation. Am J Physiol 1994; 226: H1145-H1152.

23.   Baxter GF, Goma FM, Yellon DM. Involvement of protein kinase C in the delayed cytoprotection following sublethal ischemia in rabbit myocardium. Br J Pharmacol 1995; 115: 222-224.

24.   Qiu Y, Tang X-L, Rizvi A et al. Protein kinase C mediates late preconditioning against myocardial stunning in conscious rabbits. Circulation 1996; 94 (Suppl I): I-184 (abstract).

25.   Przyklenk K, Sussman MA, Simkhovich BZ, Kloner RA. Does ischemic preconditioning trigger translocation of protein kinase C in the canine model? Circulation 1995; 92: 1546-1557.

26.   Valhaus C, Schulz R, Post H, Onallch K, Heusch A. No prevention of ischemic preconditioning by the protein kinase C inhibitor staurosporine in swine. Circ Res 1996; 79: 407-414.

27.   Ping P, Zhang J, Qiu Y et al. Ischemic preconditioning induces selective translocation of protein kinase C isoforms ε and η in the heart of conscious rabbits without subcellular redistribution of total protein kinase C activity. Circ Res 1997; 81: 404-414.

28.   Qiu Y, Ping P, Tang X-L et al. Direct evidence that protein kinase C plays an essential role in the development of late preconditioning against myocardial stunning in conscious rabbits and that ε is the isoform involved. J Clin Invest 1998 (in press).

29.   Ping P, Zhang J, Cao X et al. Ischemic preconditioning induces activation and nuclear translocation of the p44 and p42 mitogen-activated protein kinases (MAPKs) and cytosolic activation of MAPK kinases 1 and 2 (MEK 1/2) in the heart of conscious rabbits. (submitted).

30.   Ping P, Zhang J, Cao X et al. Activation of the p38 MAPK and the p46/p54 JNKs after brief episodes of ischemia/reperfusion in the heart of conscious rabbits. J Mol Cell Cardiol (abstract, in press).

31.   Ping P, Cao X, Kong D et al. PKC ε isoform induces activation of the p42/p44 MAPKs and the p46/p54 JNKs in adult rabbit cardiac myocytes. J Mol Cell Cardiol (abstract, in press).

32.   Rizvi AN, Qiu Y, Tang X-L et al. Increased synthesis of proteins is necessary for the development of late preconditioning against myocardial stunning in conscious rabbits. Circulation 1997; 96 (Suppl I): I-256 (abstract).

33.   Marber MS, Yellon DM. Myocardial adaptation, stress proteins, and the second window of protection. Ann N Y Acad Sci 1996; 793: 108-122.

34.   Marber MS, Mestril R, Chi S-H, Sayen R, Yellon DM, Dillmann WH. Overexpression of the rat inducible 70-kD heat stress protein in a transgenic mouse increases the resistance of the heart to ischemic injury. J Clin Invest 1995; 95: 1446-1456.

35.   Bolli R. Mechanism of myocardial 'stunning'. Circulation 1990; 82: 723-738.

36.   Bolli R, Jeroudi MO, Patel BS, DuBose CM, Lai EK, Roberts R, McCay PB. Direct evidence that oxygen-derived free radicals contribute to postischemic myocardial dysfunction in the intact dog. Proc Natl Acad Sci USA 1989; 86: 4695-4699.

37.   Hoshida S, Kuzuya T, Fuzi H et al. Sublethal ischemia alters myocardial antioxidant activity in canine heart. Am J Physiol 1993; 264: H33-H39.

38.   Heads RJ, Baxter GF, Latchman DS, Yellon DM. Delayed protection in rabbit heart following ischemic preconditioning is associated with modulation of HSP27 and superoxide dismutase at 24 hours. J Mol Cell Cardiol 1996; 27: A163 (abstract).

39.   Tang X-L, Qiu Y, Turrens JF, Sun J-Z, Bolli R. Late preconditioning against stunning is not mediated by increased antioxidant defenses in conscious pigs. Am J Physiol 1997; 273: H1651-H1657.

40.   Bolli R, Manchikalapudi S, Tang X-L et al. The protective effect of late preconditioning against myocardial stunning in conscious rabbits is mediated by nitric oxide synthase. Evidence that nitric oxide acts both as a trigger and as a mediator of the late phase of ischemic preconditioning. Circ Res 1997; 81: 1094-1107.

41.   Takano H, Manchikalapudi S, Tang X-L et al. Nitric oxide synthase is the mediator of late preconditioning against myocardial infarction in conscious rabbits. Circulation 1998 (in press).

3

Delayed Preconditioning Against Endothelial Dysfunction

V Richard, P Beauchamp, N Kaeffer and C Thuillez

1. Introduction

Vascular endothelial cells play an essential role in the control of vascular tone, but also in the regulation of smooth muscle cell growth, as well as of platelet and leukocyte function. Numerous experimental and clinical data suggest that these essential physiological functions of the endothelium are altered in various pathophysiological situations, such as hypertension, hypercholesterolaemia or diabetes. Such dysfunction can be characterised by an altered capacity of the endothelium to release nitric oxide (NO), associated with an increased production of oxygen-derived free radicals such as superoxide anions. A similar impairment in the endothelial synthesis of NO has also been detected at the level of the coronary circulation after myocardial ischaemia and acute or chronic reperfusion. Given the central role of NO as a vasodilating agent, but also as an inhibitor of platelet aggregation and leukocyte adhesion, it is likely that such a persistent impairment may have important deleterious consequences on the coronary arterial wall. Thus, coronary endothelium may be considered a major therapeutic target of anti-ischaemic treatments.

Recently, several experiments have suggested that preconditioning with brief periods of intermittent ischaemia, in addition to limiting infarct size, also protected coronary endothelial cells against acute or chronic reperfusion injury. Initially, much attention has been focussed on the endothelial protective effects of 'classic' preconditioning. However, recent evidence suggests the existence of a delayed phase of endothelial protection, similar to what has been reported with other aspects of ischaemia-reperfusion injury. This chapter reviews current knowledge on the existence and the possible mechanisms of such a delayed phase of endothelial protection by preconditioning.

2. Reperfusion Injury to Endothelial Cells

In the present review, we will focus on the consequences of ischaemia-reperfusion at the level of large epicardial or medium-size intramyocardial coronary arteries. Although ischaemia and reperfusion also induce major injury to the microcirculation, such microcirculatory injury is complex, involving not only endothelial cells, but also smooth muscle cells, and is probably directly related to the extent of necrosis (for example through extravascular compression and oedema leading to capillary injury and no-reflow). Thus, is is likely that any intervention which limits infarct size will ultimately result in microvascular protection. Because of this, the possible direct effects of anti-ischaemic interventions on endothelial cells may be more directly evaluated at the level of large or medium size coronary arteries, i.e. at distance from necrosis.

Evidence

Evidence that myocardial ischaemia leads to coronary endothelial dysfunction was first obtained in experiments showing that it was associated with decreased endothelium-dependent relaxation. Indeed, in 1982 (i.e. shortly after the discovery of EDRF) Ku [1] showed that ischemia was indeed associated with a decreased endothelium-dependent relaxation to thrombin. These findings were later extended to other endothelium-dependent vasodilators (such as acetylcholine) by VanBenthuysen et al [2] who also showed that this was associated in dogs with severe structural injury to endothelial cells (assessed by electron microscopy). This latter finding, which was confirmed in other species [3], suggests that this impaired endothelial function reflects actual injury to the endothelial cells, and not simply changes in endothelial function in the absence of any major structural injury, as can be the case of other diseases such as hypertension. These impaired endothelium-dependent responses after ischaemia and reperfusion are not limited to agonists such as acetylcholine, but may also be observed in response to 'physiological' stimuli for endothelium-dependant relaxations, such as for example aggregating platelets, which induce endothelium-dependent relaxations through the release of serotonin and ADP [4].

Another major feature of endothelial injury after ischaemia and reperfusion is that it is not a transient mechanism. Indeed, impaired endothelium-dependent relaxations may be prolonged at least 4 to 12

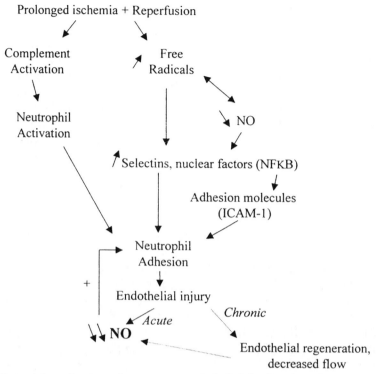

Figure 1. Potential mechanisms for coronary endothelial dysfunction after myocardial ischaemia-reperfusion

weeks after reperfusion in dogs [5] or rats 3]. In this latter species, the structural characteristics of the endothelial cells after 1 month resemble those of cells regenerated after balloon injury, a situation also characterised by chronic endothelial dysfunction [6]. Thus, it is likely that the chronically impaired endothelial function after reperfusion is a manifestation of a dysfunctional regenerated endothelium.

Mechanisms

Several studies have investigated the mechanisms of endothelial injury after ischaemia and reperfusion. First, it is important to note that most studies have reported that endothelial injury does not occur after ischaemia without reperfusion [7], suggesting that it is a manifestation of reperfusion injury. Moreover, there is a wide consensus suggesting that such reperfusion injury is mediated by reactive oxygen species which are produced during reperfusion, since this endothelial dysfunction can be attenuated or prevented by scavengers of these species [8-11]. Superoxide anions, are potent inactivators of NO [12] and also may alter endothelial binding sites for endothelium-dependent vasodilators such as acetylcholine, thus reducing the capacity of the endothelium to release NO in response to these agonists [13]. In addition, several experiments also demonstrated that reperfusion injury to the endothelium may be attenuated by interventions which limit neutrophil adhesion to endothelial cells, e.g. anti-CD18 antibodies [14] or antibodies against neutrophil adhesion molecules, such as ICAM-1 [15] or P-selectin [16]. This suggests that endothelial injury is due at least in part to neutrophils which accumulate upon reperfusion [17, 18]. Indeed, the time course of endothelial dysfunction upon reperfusion is similar to that of neutrophil accumulation [19].

Based on these findings, the following mechanisms may be advanced to explain the occurrence of endothelial injury after reperfusion (figure 1). Reperfusion after ischaemia is associated with an increased release of reactive oxygen species which trigger the rapid adhesion of neutrophils to endothelial cells. This could be due to direct activation of neutrophils by free radicals or to free radical-mediated induced expression of adhesion molecules such as selectins or ICAM-1. Increase activation or adhesion of neutrophils may also be due in part to ischaemia and/or reperfusion induced activation of complement. In parallel, free radicals may inactivate NO, which is a potent inhibitor of neutrophil activation and adhesion [20], and which may also decrease the expression of endothelial adhesion molecules [21], and this could also contribute to the increased adhesion of neutrophils. Once neutrophils have been activated, they may release free radicals and proteolytic enzymes which damage the endothelium and lead to a decreased production of NO, and this may reinforce neutrophil adhesion and endothelial injury.

Pathophysiological Significance

One critical aspect regarding the pathophysiological relevance of reperfusion-induced endothelial injury (and especially that induced at the level of large coronary arteries) is whether reperfusion exerts its deleterious effects on previously functional endothelial cells, or whether reperfusion occurs only in a context of diseased arteries with already dysfunctional endothelium, in which case prevention of reperfusion-induced endothelial injury would be of little therapeutic interest. Indeed, many risk factors for atherosclerosis, such as hypertension, diabetes, or hypercholesterolemia are known to be associated with severe endothelial dysfunction, especially at the level of the coronary circulation [22]. Furthermore, atherosclerosis also markedly impairs endothelial function [22]. However, it is important to note that atherosclerosis and the resulting endothelial dysfunction do not develop homogeneously on the coronary arterial tree. Indeed, in humans, with coronary artery diseases,

Endothelial injury (epicardial coronary arteries)

- Increased risk of vasospasm
- Increased platelet aggregation/thrombosis
- Restenosis
- Increased inflammatory response → Atherosclerosis

↓

Increased risk of infaction / reinfarction?

Figure 2. Potential consequences of reperfusion injury to coronary endothelial cells

the responses of large coronary arteries to endothelium-dependent vasodilators such as bradykinin or substance P are impaired at the side of stenosis but are preserved at the angiographically normal sites [23, 24]. Similarly, these endothelium-dependent vasodilatory responses are preserved at the spastic site in patients with vasospastic angina [25]. Thus, reperfusion injury to endothelial cells may mainly affect these non-stenotic segments of the coronary arterial tree with previously functional and viable endothelial cells. These non-stenotic segments thus represent an important target for anti-ischaemic interventions.

The potential consequences of reperfusion-induced coronary endothelial injury may be inferred from the known roles of the endothelium, and especially of endothelium-derived NO at the level of large coronary arteries (figure 2). Indeed, NO is produced constantly by large coronary arteries [26], and this permanent release of NO continuously opposes vasoconstrictor influences. Thus, an impaired release of NO may lead to an increased coronary vasoconstriction, leading to an increased risk of vasospasm. In parallel, given the role of NO and of other endothelium-derived factors such as prostacyclin as inhibitors of platelet aggregation, endothelial dysfunction after reperfusion may favor platelet aggregation and thus increase the risk for thrombosis. Finally, as mentioned before, NO is a potent inhibitor of leukocyte activation and adhesion [20] and this is true not only for neutrophils but also for monocytes [27]. Indeed, increasing evidence suggests that large artery endothelial dysfunction is one of the triggering factors for local vascular inflammatory responses which lead in the long term to the development of atherosclerosis [28]. Thus, an early and sustained impairment of endothelial function after reperfusion may have immediate consequences, for example through reinforcement of neutrophil-mediated injury, but also long term consequences, for example increased risks of vasospasm, restenosis and thrombosis and increased development of atherosclerosis.

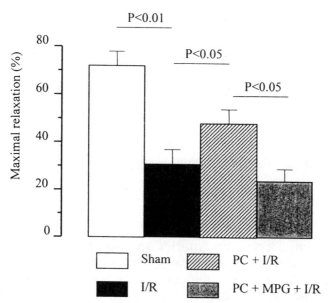

Figure 3. Prevention of reperfusion-induced coronary endothelial dysfunction by delayed preconditioning. The figure represents the maximal relaxations induced by acetylcholine in coronary artery segments isolated from sham rats, or from rats subjected to prolonged ischaemia with reperfusion (I/R) in control conditions or 24 hours after preconditioning (PC). PC was performed either in the absence or the presence of the free radical scavenger MPG. Ischaemia/reperfusion markedly reduced the response to acetylcholine, and this was partially reversed by delayed preconditioning. However, treatment by the free radical scavenger MPG abolished the protective effect of PC on endothelial function. Adapted from reference 11 with permission.

Because of this, prevention of endothelial dysfunction/injury after reperfusion, is an important therapeutic goal.

3. Evidence for Delayed Preconditioning of Coronary Endothelial Cells

Several experiments have established that 'classic' preconditioning protects coronary endothelial cells against ischaemia and reperfusion injury [7, 29, 30]. Indeed, using a rat model of ischaemia and reperfusion, we demonstrated that classic preconditioning completely prevented the impaired endothelium-dependent relaxing responses to acetylcholine assessed in vitro in coronary artery segments isolated from hearts subjected to ischaemia and acute reperfusion [7]. In this situation, the protective effect was prolonged at least 4 weeks after reperfusion [3]. However, the potential endothelial protective effects of delayed preconditioning have not been widely studied. This question has been investigated recently by our group [11]. In these experiments, anaesthetised rats were subjected to three sequences of intermittent ischaemia and allowed to recover. Twenty four hours later, rats were re-anaesthetised and subjected to a standard ischaemia-reperfusion protocol, i.e. 20 minutes of ischaemia and 60 minutes of reperfusion. At the end of the reperfusion period, the heart was removed, the left (ischaemic) coronary artery was dissected and a 1.5-2 mm long segment was taken distal to the site of occlusion and mounted in a small vessel myograph for isometric tension recording. The main result of this study is shown in figure 3. As shown on this figure, as compared to sham-operated animals, the response to acetylcholine was markedly reduced in arteries taken from animals subjected to ischaemia-reperfusion, and this was partly prevented by late preconditioning. Thus, this finding suggests that late preconditioning, in addition to its beneficial effects on infarct size and postischaemic myocardial contractile dysfunction, also protects coronary endothelial cells against ischaemia and reperfusion injury.

In addition to brief ischaemia, other interventions have been shown to induced delayed cardioprotection, for example heat stress. Indeed, in other experiments, we also demonstrated that prior heat stress, in addition to limiting infarct size, also completely prevented reperfusion-induced endothelial dysfunction [31].

4. Mechanisms of Delayed Protection

One important question regarding the mechanisms of delayed endothelial protection by preconditioning is whether this is a direct effect or whether endothelial protection occurs simply secondary to myocardial protection. However, as represented in figure 4 which regroups several interventions in which infarct size and endothelial dysfunction were measured in parallel, there appears to be a marked dissociation between the extent of necrosis and the severity of dysfunction. For example, despite the fact that classic preconditioning induces an effect on infarct size which is much more marked than that of heat stress, both interventions induce a similar degree of endothelial protection. Similarly, in our experiments, heat stress and delayed preconditioning induce similar decreases in infarct size, but the effect of heat stress on endothelial function was more marked than that of delayed preconditioning. Finally, in our rat model, free radical scavengers such as mercaptopropionylglycine (MPG) completely prevent reperfusion-induced endothelial dysfunction but do not affect infarct size. Taken together, these observations demonstrate that there is no relationship between infarct size and the extent of endothelial dysfunction, and suggest that the endothelial protection induced by interventions such as delayed preconditioning is a direct effect, and is not secondary to their effects on the cardiac myocytes. However, several similarities may exist

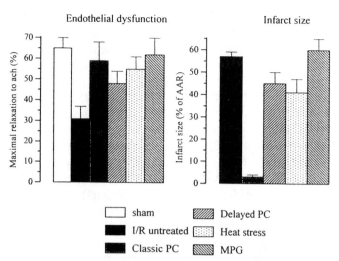

Figure 4. Dissociation between the endothelial protective effects (left) and the infarct size limiting effects of various interventions in the rat model of ischaemia-reperfusion. Note that 1) heat stress and classic preconditioning induce similar degrees of endothelial protection but markedly different effects on infarct size; 2) the effect of heat stress on endothelial function is more marked than that of delayed preconditioning but their effect on infarct size is similar; 3) MPG completely prevents reperfusion-induced endothelial dysfunction but does not affect infarct size. Thus, there appears to be no relationship between the endothelial protection and the infarct size limitation induced by these various interventions.

between the mechanisms of the myocardial and the endothelial protective effects, both in terms of triggers and in terms of mediators of the protective effects.

5. Mediators of Protection

As mentioned before, it is now well accepted that reperfusion-induced endothelial injury is mediated by oxygen-derived free radicals. Thus, it is tempting to speculate that delayed preconditioning somehow reduces the production of free radicals during reperfusion, for example by increasing the cell's antioxidant defences. Indeed, brief ischaemia may increase the activity of antioxidant enzymes such as superoxide dismutase (SOD), catalase or glutathione peroxidase in isolated myocytes [32, 33], and in vivo [34-37] although such an effect was not found in all experiments [38]. Moreover, prevention of the increase in SOD activity by an antisense oligonucleotide corresponding to the initiation chain of SOD abolished the protective effect of late preconditioning against hypoxia in isolated myocytes [32]. Thus, such an increase in antioxidant activity represents a likely mechanism by which preconditioning induces endothelial protection (see Chapter 8).

Another mechanism by which delayed preconditioning may protect the endothelium is though an increased production of NO during ischaemia and reperfusion. Indeed, we and others have shown that addition of exogenous NO or stimulation of endogenous production of this factor during ischaemia and reperfusion results in a marked endothelial protection [39-41]. Given the known roles of NO, it is likely that this endothelial protective effect is due either to an increased inactivation of free radicals [12] and/or a decreased adhesion of leukocytes, possibly in part through a decreased expression of nuclear factors such as NFκB, leading to a decreased expression of endothelial adhesion molecules.

Major (although indirect) support for the hypothesis of a role of an increased production of NO by delayed preconditioning comes from experiments, in which the effect on coronary endothelial function of a brief (10 minute) coronary occlusion followed by prolonged (5 day) reperfusion was studied in conscious, chronically instrumented dogs [42]. In these experiments, it was demonstrated that brief ischaemia was associated with a delayed increase in the coronary flow response to two endothelium-dependent vasodilators, acetylcholine and bradykinin (figure 5). In these experiments, endothelium-dependent responses started to increase after 6 hours of reperfusion, peaked after 1-2 days and returned to baseline over the next 4 days. These increased functional responses were accompanied by an increased production of NO, as estimated by measurement of the coronary arteriovenous differences in nitrates and nitrites (figure 5). Thus, although these experiments do not address the possible role of NO in delayed preconditioning, they clearly demonstrate that brief periods of ischaemia do result in a delayed enhanced production of NO, and that the time course of this increase in compatible with a role in delayed preconditioning against endothelial injury.

Recently, we have investigated whether heat stress also increases NO production in normal rats arteries [43]. In these experiments, we found that heat stress indeed induced a delayed (24 hours) increase in NO-dependent relaxations at the level of the aorta, the mesenteric and the coronary arteries (assessed in vitro). Thus, as in the case of brief ischaemia, the time course of the increased NO release is compatible with a role of this factor in the delayed protective effect of heat stress.

Finally, as in the case of myocardial protection, it is possible that the delayed endothelial protection by preconditioning may be mediated by the expression of stress proteins such as heat shock proteins (HSPs). Indeed, endothelial cells may express HSP70 [44, 45] and preliminary experiments suggest that transfection of cultured endothelial cells with HSP70 renders those cells more resistant to hypoxia [46]. However, to our knowledge, no experiments have evaluated the direct role of HSP in the delayed endothelial protection induced by preconditioning.

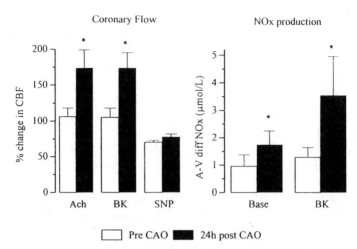

Figure 5. Delayed (24 hours) increase in NO production after brief (10 minute) coronary artery occlusion (CAO) in conscious dogs. CAO induced a delayed increase in the coronary blood flow (CBF) response to the endothelium-dependent vasodilators acetylcholine (Ach) and bradykinin (BK), without affecting the endothelium-independent response to the NO donor sodium nitroprusside (SNP). In parallel CAO induced a delayed increase in basal and BK-induced release of NO, as indicated by increased arteriovenous production of nitrates and nitrites. From reference 42 with permission.

6. Triggers of Protection

As mentioned above, the delayed protection induced by preconditioning is probably mediated by an increased production of NO during prolonged ischaemia and reperfusion, together with a decrease production of free radicals during reperfusion. Several experiments suggest that changes in free radicals and/or NO production may also act as triggers for these delayed changes after preconditioning.

We found that administration of the free radical scavenger MPG abolished the endothelial protective effects of preconditioning (figure 3). This is similar to what has already been demonstrated in a pig model of myocardial stunning [47] and suggests that oxidative stress induced by reperfusion after preconditioning is necessary for the development of the protective mechanisms leading to endothelial protection, possibly through an increased expression of antioxidant enzymes or NOS. Indeed, oxidant stress induces a delayed increase in the activity of antioxidant enzymes in endothelial cells [44]. Thus, one likely explanation for our results is that oxidative stress induced by preconditioning induces a delayed increase in antioxidant activity in myocytes and/or endothelial cells, and this in turn protects the endothelial cells against further, more severe oxidative stress during reperfusion after prolonged ischaemia.

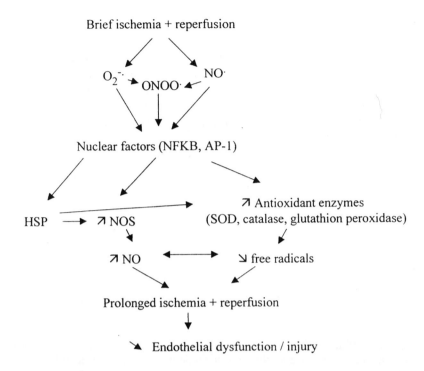

Figure 6. Potential mechanisms for the delayed coronary endothelial protective effects of preconditioning

Indirect evidence also exists for a role of NO as a trigger for late protection. Indeed, in conscious dogs, inhibition of NO synthesis during brief ischemia blocks the delayed enhanced endothelium-dependent vasodilatation (figure 5) [42]. Interestingly, NO may also act as a trigger for the delayed protective effects of preconditioning, against stunning [48] (see Chapter 2) and may also contribute to its effect on infarct size [49]. Taken together, this suggests that (as in the case of stunning), the development of delayed endothelial protection by preconditioning may be mediated both by free radicals and NO. One possibility to explain this dual role is that superoxide anions and NO react to product other radical intermediates such as peroxynitrites [50], resulting in an early oxidative stress which could be responsible for the synthesis of various proteins (such as antioxidant enzymes, NO synthase or HSPs) responsible for the endothelial protective effects.

7. Conclusion

In addition to exerting myocardial protective effects, delayed preconditioning also protects coronary endothelial cells against reperfusion injury. Given the various known roles of these cells, such an endothelial protective effect may translate into decreased risks of vasospasm, platelet aggregation and atherosclerosis. Identification of the mechanisms responsible for the endogenous protective effect of delayed preconditioning may lead to the development of new pharmacological interventions which could protect the endothelium during reperfusion, but also in other disease states also characterised by increased oxidative stress, such as hypertension [51], hypercholesterolaemia [52] or atherosclerosis [53].

References

1.   Ku DD. Coronary vascular reactivity after acute myocardial infarction. Science 1982; 218: 576-578.

2.   VanBenthuysen KM, McMurtry IF, Horwitz LD. Reperfusion after coronary occlusion in dogs impairs endothelium-dependent relaxation to acetylcholine and augments contractile reactivity in vitro. J Clin Invest 1987; 79: 265-274.

3.   Kaeffer N, Richard V, Henry JP, Thuillez C. Preconditioning prevents chronic reperfusion-induced coronary endothelial dysfunction in rats. Am J Physiol. 1996; 271: H842-H849.

4.   Pearson PJ, Schaff HV, Vanhoutte PM. Acute impairment of endothelium-dependent relaxations to aggregating platelets following reperfusion injury in canine coronary arteries. Circ Res 1990; 67: 385-393.

5.   Pearson PJ, Schaff HV, Vanhoutte PM. Long-term impairment of endothelium-dependent relaxations to aggregating platelets after reperfusion injury in canine coronary arteries. Circulation 1990; 81: 1921-1927.

6.   Shimokawa H, Aarhus LL, Vanhoutte PM. Porcine coronary arteries with regenerated endothelium have a reduced endothelium-dependent responsiveness to aggregating platelets and serotonin. Circ Res 1987; 61: 256-270.

7.   Richard V, Kaeffer N, Tron C, Thuillez C. Ischemic preconditioning protects against coronary endothelial dysfunction induced by ischemia and reperfusion. Circulation 1994; 89: 1254-1261.

8.   Tsao PS, Aoki N, Lefer DJ, Johnson III G, Lefer AM. Time course of endothelium dysfonction and myocardial injury during myocardial ischemia and reperfusion in the cat. Circulation 1990; 82: 1402-1412.

9.   Gross GJ, O'Rourke ST, Pelc LR. Myocardial and endothelial dysfunction after multiple, brief coronary occlusions : role of oxygen radicals. Am J Physiol 1992; 263: H1703-H1709.

10.   Mehta JL, Nichols WW, Donnelly WH et al. Protection by superoxide dismutase from myocardial dysfunction and attenuation of vasodilator reserve after coronary occlusion and reperfusion in dog. Circ Res 1989; 65: 1283-1295.

11.   Kaeffer N, Richard V, Thuillez C. Delayed coronary endothelial protection 24 hours after preconditioning. Role of free radicals. Circulation 1997; 96: 2311-2316.

12.   Gryglewski RJ, Palmer RMJ, Moncada S. Superoxide anion is involved in the breakdown of endothelium-derived relaxing factor. Nature 1986; 320: 454-460.

13.   Pieper GM, Gross GJ. Selective impairment of endothelium-dependent relaxation by oxygen-derived free radicals: distinction between receptor versus non receptor mediators. Blood Vessels 1989; 26: 44-47.

14.   Ma XL, Tsao PS, Lefer AM. Antibody to CD-18 exerts endothelial and cardiac protective effects in myocardial ischemia and reperfusion. J Clin Invest 1995; 88: 1237-1243.

15.   Ma XL, Lefer DJ, Lefer AM, Rothlein R. Coronary endothelial and cardiac protective effects of a monoclonal antibody to intercellular adhesion molecule-1 in myocardial ischemia and reperfusion. Circulation 1992; 86: 937-946.

16.   Weyrich AS, Ma XY, Lefer DJ, Albertine KH, Lefer AM. In vivo neutralization of P-selectin protects feline heart and endothelium in myocardial ischemia and reperfusion injury. J Clin Invest 1993; 91: 2620-2629.

17.   Go LO, Murry CE, Richard V, Weischedel GR, Jennings RB, Reimer KA. Myocardial neutrophil accumulation during reperfusion after reversible and irreversible ischemic injury. Am J Physiol 1988; 255: H1188-H1198.

18.   Kloner RA, Giacomelli F, Alker KJ, Hale SL, Matthews R, Bellow S. Influx of neutrophils into the walls of large epicardial coronary arteries in response to ischemia/reperfusion. Circulation 1991; 84: 1758-1772.

19.   Tsao PS, Aoki N, Lefer DJ, Johnson III G, Lefer AM. Time course of endothelium dysfonction and myocardial injury during myocardial ischemia and reperfusion in the cat. Circulation 1990; 82: 1402-1412.

20.   Kubes P, Suzuki M, Granger DN. Nitric oxide: an endogenous modulator of leukocyte adhesion. Proc Natl Acad Sci USA 1991; 88: 4651-4655.

21.   De Caterina R, Libby P, Peng H-B et al. Nitric oxide decreases cytokine-induced endothelial activation. Nitric oxide selectively reduces endothelial expression of adhesion molecules and proinflammatory cytokines. J Clin Invest 1995; 96: 60-68.

22.   Luscher TF, Richard V, Tschudi M, Yang Z, Boulanger C. Endothelial control of vascular tone in large and small coronary arteries. J Am Coll Cardiol 1990; 15: 519-527.

23.   Kuga T, Egashira K, Mohri M et al. Bradykinin-induced vasodilation is impaired at the atherosclerotic site but is preserved at the spastic site of human coronary arteries in vivo. Circulation 1995; 92: 183-189.

24.   Crossman DC, Larkin SW, Dashwook MR, Davies GJ, Yacoub M, Maseri A. Responses of atherosclerotic human coronary arteries in vivo to the endothelium-dependent vasodilator substance P. Circulation 1991; 84: 2001-2010.

25.   Egashira K, Inou T, Yamada A, Hirooka Y, Takeshita A. Preserved endothelium-dependent vasodilation at the vasospastic site in patients with variant angina. J Clin Invest 1992; 89: 1047-1052.

26.   Chu A, Chambers DE, Lin C-C et al. Effects of inhibition of nitric oxide formation on basal vasomotion and endothelium-dependent responses of the coronary arteries in awake dogs. J Clin Invest 1991; 87: 1964-1968.

27.   Tsao PS, Buitrago R, Chan JR, Cooke JP. Fluid flow inhibits endothelial adhesiveness. Nitric oxide and transcriptional regulation of VCAM-1. Circulation 1996; 94: 1682-1689.

28.   Ross R: The pathogenesis of atherosclerosis: a perspective for the 1990s. Nature 1993; 362: 801-809.

29.   DeFily DV, Chillian WM. Preconditioning protects coronary arteriolar endothelium against ischemia - reperfusion injury. Am J Physiol 1993; 265: H700-H706.

30.   Bouchard JF, Lamontagne D. Mechanisms of protection afforded by preconditioning to endothelial function against ischemic injury. Am J Physiol 1996, 271: H1801-1806.

31.   Kaeffer N, Richard V, Thuillez C. Heat stress protects coronary against coronary endothelial dysfunction after myocardial ischemia and reperfusion in rats. Circulation 1995; 92:I-653 (Abstract)

32.   Yamashita N, Nishida M, Hoshida S et al. Induction of manganese superoxide dismutase in rat cardiac myocytes increases tolerance to hypoxia 24 hours after preconditioning. J Clin Invest 1994; 94: 2193-2199.

33.   Zhou X, Zhai X, Ashraf M. Direct evidence that initial oxidative stress triggered by preconditioning contributes to second window of protection by endogenous antioxidant enzyme in myocytes. Circulation 1996; 93: 1177-1184.

34.   Das DK, Engelman RM, Kimura Y. Molecular adaptation of cellular defences following preconditioning of the heart by repeated ischaemia. Cardiovasc Res 1993: 27: 578-584.

35.   Das DK, Prasad MR, Tu D, Jones RM. Preconditioning of heart by repeated stunning. Adaptive modification of antioxidative defense system. J Mol Cell Cardiol. 1992; 38: 739-749.

36.   Hoshida S, Kuzuya T, Fuji H et al. Sublethal ischemia alters myocardial antioxidant activity in canine heart. Am J Physiol. 1993; 264: H33-H39.

37.   Steeves G, Singh N, Singal PK. Preconditioning and antioxidant defense against reperfusion injury. Ann N Y Acad Sci. 1994; 723: 116-127.

38.   Turrens JF, Thornton J, Barnard ML, Snyder S, Liu G, Downey JM. Protection from reperfusion injury by preconditioning heart does not involve increased antioxidant defenses. Am J Physiol 1992; 262: H585-H589.

39.   Richard V, Blanc T, Kaeffer N, Tron C, Thuillez C. Myocardial and coronary endothelial protective effects of acetylcholine after myocardial ischemia and reperfusion in rats. Role of nitric oxide. Br J Pharmacol 1995; 115: 1532-1538.

40.   Ma XL, Weyrich AS, Lefer DJ, Lefer AM. Diminished basal nitric oxide release after myocardial ischemia and reperfusion promotes neutrophil adherence to coronary endothelium. Circ Res 1993; 72: 403-412.

41.   Weyrich AS, Ma XL, Lefer AM. The role of L-arginine in ameliorating reperfusion injury after myocardial ischemia in the cat. Circulation 1992; 86: 279-288.

42.   Kim SJ, Ghaleh B, Kudej RK, Huang CH, Hintze TH, Vatner SF. Delayed enhanced nitric oxide-mediated coronary vasodilation following brief ischemia and prolonged reperfusion in concious dogs. Circ Res 1997; 81: 53-59.

43.   Richard V, JP Henry, C Artigues, N Kaeffer, C Thuillez. Prior heat stress increases NO-dependent relaxations in isolated rat arteries. Circulation 1997: 96:I-349 (Abstract)

44.   Lu D, Maulik N, Moraru II, Kreutzer DL, Das DK. Molecular adaptation of vascular endothelial cells to oxidative stress. Am J Physiol 1993; 264: C715-C722.

45.   Aucoin MM, Barhoumi R, Kochevar DT, Granger HJ, Burghardt RC. Oxidative injury of coronary venular endothelial cells depletes intracellular glutathione and induces HSP 70 mRNA. Am J Physiol 1995; 268: H1651-H1658.

46.   Suzuki K, Bai H, Kadoba K, Shirakura R. Heat shock protein 70 overexpressed by gene transfection enhances the tolerance to ischemia not only in cardiomyocytes but also in coronary endothelial cells. Circulation 1995; 92: I-653 (Abstract)

47.   Sun JZ, Tang XL, Park SW, Qiu Y, Turrens JF, Bolli R. Evidence for an essential role of reactive oxygen species in the genesis of late preconditioning against myocardial stunning in conscious pigs. J Clin Invest 1996; 97: 562-576.

48.   Bolli R, Batti Z, Tang XL et al. Evidence that late preconditioning against myocardial stunning in conscious rabbits is triggered by the generation of nitric oxide. Circ Res 1997; 81: 42-52.

49.   Qiu Y, Rizvi A, Tang XL et al. Nitric oxide triggers late preconditioning against myocardial infarction in conscious rabbits. Am J Physiol 1997; 273: H2931-H2936.

50.   Beckman JS, Beckman TW, Chen J, Marshall PA, Freeman BA. Apparent hydroxyl radical production by peroxynitrite: implication for endothelial injury from nitric oxide and superoxide. Proc Natl Acad Sci USA 1990; 87: 1620-1624.

51.   Alexander RW. Hypertension and the pathogenesis of atherosclerosis. Oxidative stress and the mediation of arterial inflammatory response : a new perspective. Hypertension 1995; 25: 155-161.

52.   Ohara Y, Peterson TE, Harrison DG. Hypercholesterolemia increases endothelial superoxide anion production. J Clin Invest 1993; 91: 2546-2551.

53.   Harrison DG, Ohara Y. Physiological consequences of increased vascular oxidant stresses in hypercholesterolemia and atherosclerosis; implications for impaired vasomotion. Am J Cardiol 1995; 75: 75B-81B.

4

Delayed Preconditioning Against Ventricular Arrhythmias

A Vegh and J R Parratt

1. Introduction

In 1989, not long after the first description of the preconditioning phenomenon by Murry et al. [1], demonstrating a protective effect against myocardial ischaemic damage (infarct size limitation), we explored the possibility that preconditioning could also protect the heart against those severe ventricular arrhythmias which arise soon after the onset of myocardial ischaemia. We were particularly interested to assess the extent to which the coronary endothelium determines arrhythmia severity following coronary artery occlusion and whether this plays a role in ischaemic preconditioning. In this chapter, we describe the protection against ventricular arrhythmias afforded by preconditioning, with particular emphasis on the delayed form of protection.

2. Experimental Background

Most of this work was performed in the Department of Pharmacology in Szeged where an experimental model of myocardial ischaemia-reperfusion in dogs has been long established. The model is that of acute coronary artery occlusion in dogs, anaesthetised either with a barbiturate or, more commonly, a mixture of chloralose and urethane. Ventricular arrhythmias following coronary artery occlusion are less pronounced in animals anaesthetised with barbiturates than they are with certain other anaesthetics. Large dogs are used, in excess of 17 kg, because arrhythmia severity depends in part on heart size; ventricular fibrillation (VF) is rare

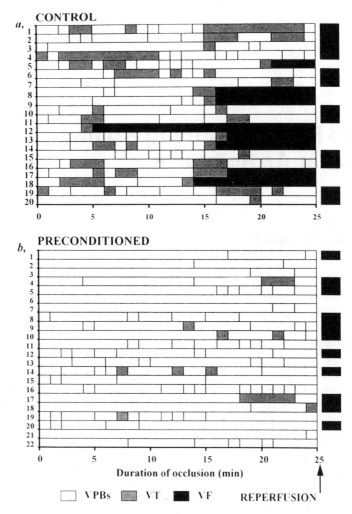

Figure 1. Panel a. Ventricular arrhythmias in 20 open-chest anaesthetised dogs subjected to LAD occlusion for 25 minutes, followed by sudden reperfusion. All dogs exhibited VPBs and there is some evidence that these occur in two phases, phase 1a (between 0 and 10 minutes) and phase 1b (between 15 and 25 minute). When VF occurred during occlusion it was always preceded by a brief period of VT. All dogs succumbed to VF either during occlusion (n=8) or reperfusion (n=12). **Panel b.** Ventricular arrhythmias in 22 dogs subjected to ischaemic preconditioning by two 5 minute periods of coronary artery occlusion terminating 20 minutes prior to a 25 minute occlusion of the LAD. The severity of ventricular arrhythmias is markedly reduced by preconditioning; no dog fibrillated during occlusion and there were occasional periods of VT in only 7 of the 22 dogs. Survival from the combined ischaemia-reperfusion insult was markedly increased by preconditioning from 0 % (in control dogs) to 50 % in the preconditioned group.

in dogs with a body weight of less than 16 or 17 kg [2]. There is a marked variation in the severity of ventricular arrhythmias in mongrel dogs subjected to coronary artery occlusion and this necessitates using relatively large group sizes. In our own experience a group size of around 10 dogs is minimal for the assessement of, for example, substances with potential antiarrhythmic activity. Arrhythmia severity is assessed by evaluating the incidences of VF and ventricular tachycardia (VT), the duration and number of episodes of VT and the number of ventricular premature beats (VPBs) which occur during the occlusion period. The extent and degree of ischaemia is monitored by epicardial ST-segment mapping and by measurements of the degree of inhomogeneity of electrical activation within the area supplied by the occluded artery, which we regard as perhaps the best index of ischaemia severity [3, 4].

The variation in arrhythmia severity following coronary artery occlusion in normal dogs is illustrated in Figure 1a. It shows that, in a series of 20 dogs, VF occurred during the occlusion period in eight; in every case this was preceded by a brief period of VT. The figure also shows that ventricular arrhythmias, and particularly VT, occur in two distinct phases during the occlusion period. In 12 dogs there was a period of VT within the first six or seven minutes; this was followed by a relatively quiet phase between 10 and 15 minutes, followed by a later phase in which VT and VF were common. These two distinct phases have been referred to as phase 1a and phase 1b respectively; the mechanisms of these two particular phases of potentially life-threatening arrhythmias appear to be different [5]. The other conclusion from this figure is that those dogs that survived the occlusion succumbed to VF following reperfusion at the end of the occlusion period. VF thus occurred in all of these 20 control dogs subjected to coronary artery occlusion. These and other studies [6] suggest that VF, arising from reperfusion of the ischaemic myocardium, could lead to sudden cardiac death in the clinical situation. One could visualise that in patients with a narrowed coronary artery, the complete occlusion of that vessel by a thrombus at a site of endothelial dysfunction and by its later disintegration, might result in sudden reperfusion of the previously ischaemic area of the ventricular wall. The resultant electrical instability would then lead to VF. How frequently this occurs in patients who die suddenly is difficult to document but it could be a major contributory factor [17].

3. From Early to Delayed Protection

In this canine model, ischaemic preconditioning results in a marked suppression of ventricular arrhythmias (Figure 1b). The preconditioning stimulus in these studies was two 5 minute periods of coronary artery occlusion terminating 20 minutes before the prolonged (25 minute)

occlusion of the same coronary artery. The most striking effect illustrated
in this figure is that in these 22 preconditioned dogs no VF occurred
during the prolonged period of ischaemia. The distribution of ectopic
beats during the occlusion period was similar to that in the control dogs
but the number of VPBs was much reduced. Only six of the 22 dogs
exhibited VT and this was of short duration. Further, half of the
preconditioned dogs survived reperfusion. These results clearly indicate
that, in this canine model, preconditioning by short coronary artery
occlusions markedly reduces the severity of ventricular arrhythmias that
occur during a longer period of ischaemia and increases survival from a
combined ischaemia-reperfusion insult [4].

There is increasing evidence to suggest that similar protection
against ventricular arrhythmias could also occur in humans [8]. Tamura
and colleagues [9] showed that severe angina within 24 hours of onset of
acute myocardial infarction reduces the occurrence of life-threatening
ventricular tachyarrhythmias, mainly associated with reperfusion, during
successful reperfusion therapy. Similar results have been found in
patients who underwent coronary angioplasty [10] where a preceding
vessel occlusion-reperfusion cycle of brief duration increased the electrical
stability of the ischaemic myocardium. Compared to the first occlusion,
the number of VPBs was reduced during the second occlusion without
any significant difference in the signs of myocardial ischaemia or in the
haemodynamic variables between sequential occlusions [10].

4. Delayed Protection Against Arrhythmias by Cardiac Pacing

In 1993, Kuzuya and colleagues [11] showed in dogs, and Marber and
colleagues [12] in rabbits, that preconditioning with four 5 minute
coronary artery occlusions, 24 hours before sustained ischaemia, resulted
in marked reduction in infarct size compared to the unpreconditioned
controls. This phenomenon which has been confirmed on many
occasions and in a variety of experimental model is now known as
'delayed' or 'second window' preconditioning [13]. The first attempt to
determine, whether delayed protection exists against ventricular
arrhythmias was made in 1994 [14, 15]. We knew from our previous
studies that rapid cardiac pacing protects the heart against the effects of a
subsequent coronary artery occlusion [16, 17]. Indeed, protection against
ischaemia-induced ventricular arrhythmias by pacing was as marked as it
is when induced by brief coronary artery occlusions although the duration
of protection is shorter [17]. We supposed that cardiac pacing would be a
better stimulus for preconditioning than transient coronary artery
occlusions since the introduction of a pacing electrode into the right
ventricle does not require extensive surgery, such as thoracotomy. This

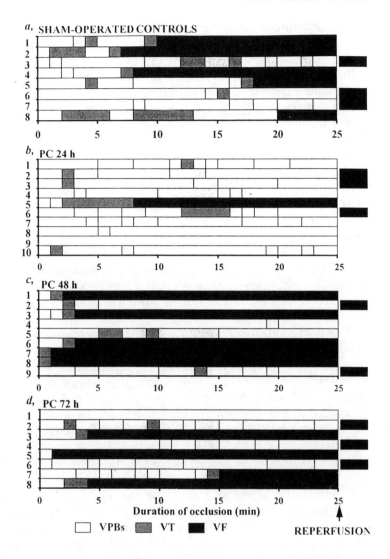

Figure 2. Time course of delayed protection against ischaemia-reperfusion induced ventricular arrhythmias resulting from brief periods of cardiac pacing. The figure illustrates the severity of ventricular arrhythmias during a 25 minute occlusion and reperfusion of the LAD coronary artery in sham-operated control dogs (a) and in dogs subjected to right ventricular pacing (four times for 5 minutes, at a pacing rate of 220 beats per minute), 24 hours (b), 48 hours (c) and 72 hours (d) previously.

method would also minimise the effect of those mediators which are released by surgical trauma and postoperative inflammation and which could influence the generation and severity of ventricular arrhythmias.

In these studies, dogs were lightly anaesthetised with pentobarbitone and a pacing electrode placed in the right ventricle. The dogs were then paced, at a rate of 220 beats per minute for four 5 minute periods, with 5 minute rest ("reperfusion") periods between the pacing stimuli. Sham-operated dogs served as contols; in these the pacing electrode was introduced into the right ventricle but the dogs were not paced. At various times after the pacing stimulus (24, 48 and 72 hours) the dogs were re-anaesthetised with a mixture of chloralose and urethane, thoracotomised and the anterior descending branch of the left coronary artery (LAD) occluded for 25 minutes. The ischaemic myocardium was then reperfused [17].

Figure 2 illustrates the time course of delayed protection against ischaemia and reperfusion-induced ventricular arrhythmias resulting from cardiac pacing. In the sham-operated controls occlusion of the LAD resulted in severe ventricular arrhythmias similar to those seen in those control dogs illustrated in figure 1. There were large numbers of VPBs and many VT episodes during occlusion and 63% of these dogs fibrillated during the occlusion period (Figure 2a). Furthermore, no dog in the sham control group survived the combined ischaemia-reperfusion insult (Figure 2a). When dogs were paced and 24 hours afterwards subjected to coronary artery occlusion there was a pronounced reduction in the severity of ventricular arrhythmias. Compared to the sham-operated controls, the number of VPBs (145 ± 20 vs. 583 ± 62, $P < 0.05$) and the number of episodes of VT (3.5 ± 3.1 vs. 9.4 ± 5.4; $P < 0.05$) during occlusion were significantly reduced, as were the incidences of these arrhythmias. In contrast to the controls, the incidence of occlusion-induced VF was only 10%, and 60% of these dogs survived the occlusion-reperfusion insult. The protection appeared to be attenuated when the time interval between the pacing stimulus and the coronary artery occlusion was extended to 48 or 72 hours (Figure 2 c and d). Although the number of VPBs and VT episodes remained low in those dogs that survived the occlusion, the incidence of VF during occlusion was again increased if the time interval between the pacing stimulus and the occlusion was prolonged to 48 hours (56% incidence) or 72 hours (50%). Thus, the overall survival in these groups was 22% and 13%, respectively, values not significantly different from those in sham-operated controls.

We do not understand precisely why cardiac pacing protects the heart against the effects of a subsequent coronary artery occlusion. A reasonable explanation for the protection would be the increase in myocardial oxygen demand as a result of increased heart rate and wall stress, coupled with a reduced blood flow to the subendocardium due, in part at least, to the elevated left ventricular filling pressure [17]. Certainly, rapid cardiac pacing in a conscious rabbit model results in ischaemia-induced electrocardiographic changes and alterations in left ventricular filling pressure [18]. What is also debatable is whether the reduction in arrhythmia severity following cardiac pacing is due to a reduction in ischaemic damage (infarct size) or whether the mechanisms underlying these two endpoints are different. Our studies made no attempt to determine whether cardiac pacing reduces infarct size, although both epicardial ST-segment elevation and the degree of inhomogeneity of electrical activation measured within the ischaemic area during occlusion (indices of ischaemia severity), are reduced in parallel with the reduction in the number of VPBs during occlusion (Figure 3). One of the possible explanations for the reduction of arrhythmia severity following cardiac pacing is a reduction in the severity of ischaemia during coronary artery occlusion. However, the severity of ischaemia, for which we have only imprecise measurements, is just one factor responsible for life-threatening ventricular arrhythmias following coronary artery occlusion. Others would certainly include catecholamine and thromboxane release, potassium loss, myocardial temperature and platelet activation, none of which are directly related to ischaemia severity.

5. Time Course and Renewal of Delayed Protection

Of particular interest is the fact that the time course of delayed protection against arrhythmias is rather similar to that recently described against stunning in a porcine model of delayed preconditioning [19, 20] (see chapter 2), and against infarction in rabbits [21, 22] (see chapter 1). For example, delayed protection against ischaemic damage in the rabbit extended over a three day period [21, 22]. In this model, the most marked infarct limitation effect was observed 48 and 72 hours after preconditioning; 96 hours after the preconditioning stimulus no protection against infarction was seen (see Chapter 1). Similarly, protection against stunning was most marked 24 and 72 hours after preconditioning and disappeared within six days of the preconditioning stimulus [20]. In these studies protection against infarction and stunning was somewhat more prolonged than against arrhythmias in our canine model in which a different form of preconditioning stimulus was used. The variation in the time course of protection against ischaemic damage, stunning and ventricular arrhythmias might be explained by species and endpoint differences, or by the assumption that the delayed protection is weaker than the early protective effect of the same preconditioning stimulus [23]. More likely it results from a difference in the nature of the preconditioning stimulus. Perhaps cardiac pacing is a less powerful stimulus for inducing

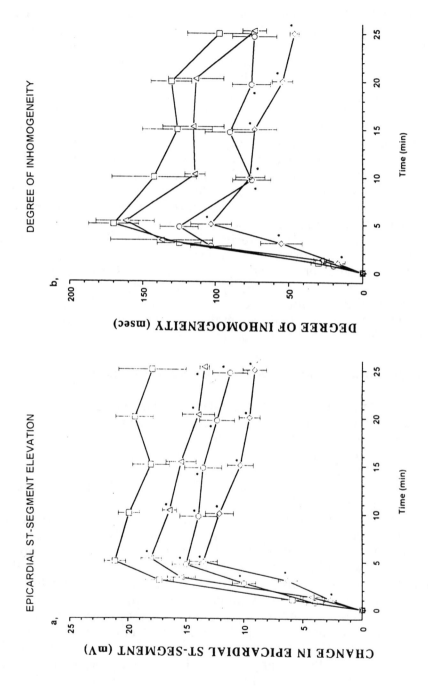

Figure 3 (opposite). Changes in epicardial ST-segment elevation (**Panel a**) and in the degree of inhomogeneity of electrical activation (**Panel b**) during a 25 minute occlusion of a coronary artery in sham-operated control dogs (open squares, n = 8) and in dogs subjected to cardiac pacing 24 hours (open diamonds, n = 10), 48 hours (open circles, n = 9) or 72 hours (open triangles, n =8) previously. *P < 0.05 vs. sham-operated controls.

protection than is brief, and complete, coronary artery occlusion. Although we know little about the optimal conditions required for this delayed protection against arrhythmias by cardiac pacing, we do know that if the pacing stimulus is repeated at a time when the protective effects of the previous pacing have faded then the protection against arrhythmias is even more prolonged and can last for days [24, 25]. This time course is then similar to the protection against ischaemic damage induced by short coronary artery occlusions [21, 22].

In these experiments we paced dogs on day one under light pentobarbitone anaesthesia, but instead of occluding the coronary artery on day three, when the protection from a single pacing stimulus is virtually lost, we repeated the pacing stimulus. Forty eight, 72 and 96 hours after this second pacing stimulus we re-anaesthetised the dogs and occluded the LAD for 25 minutes. Repeated pacing at a time when protection from a single pacing period had already faded resulted in a more marked and prolonged protection than when dogs were paced only once. Thus, at this time, the most marked protection against fibrillation occurred 48 and 72 hours after the second pacing stimulus. The protection was lost by 96 hours [24, 25].

These experiments raise the possibility that the myocardium can be maintained in a continuous preconditioned state by repeating the preconditioning stimulus. Such a preconditioning stimulus might be regular physical exercise (reviewed recently in reference 26). In an interesting study Hull and colleagues [27] showed that in dogs following 6 weeks treadmill exercise training the repetitive extrasystole threshold was increased by 44% and there was no VF during acute myocardial ischaemia. Although the precise mechanisms by which exercise protects the myocardium against ventricular arrhythmias is not known, it might well be that a shift in autonomic balance characterised by increased vagal tone [27] or increased release of nitric oxide (NO) from the endothelial cells [28] are involved. It is also not clear what intensity of exercise is required to induce this protection. Severe exercise can also trigger a cardiac event [29]. However, it does seem likely that regular exercise can reduce the risk of infarction and sudden cardiac death [30, 31] by mechanisms still to be clarified. (See also Chapter 8.)

6. Delayed Protection Against Arrhythmias Induced by Prostacyclin

The concept of delayed cardioprotection by drugs was pioneered by Laszlo Szekeres in Szeged. In the early 1980s he and his colleagues showed that the administration of 7-oxo-prostacyclin, a stable derivative of prostacyclin, in a variety of species (dogs, rats, cats, guinea pigs and rabbits) resulted in what was described as a 'late appearing, long lasting' cardioprotection. This had a time course similar to that described several years later for the delayed effect of ischaemic peconditioning and of cardiac pacing [32]. The protection induced by 7-oxo-prostacyclin depended on protein synthesis and was manifested in a variety of ways, including enhanced recovery of contractile function following a period of ischaemia and reperfusion, protection against the calcium paradox and the ultrastructural changes resulting from global ischaemia and, last but not least, protection against ischaemia and reperfusion-induced ventricular arrhythmias (reviewed in references 33 and 34).

7. Delayed Protection Against Arrhythmias Induced by Endotoxins

Another, more recent, example of delayed cardioprotection by an acute intervention are studies with bacterial endotoxin (lipopolysaccharide, LPS). It has long been known that endotoxin, such as that derived from *Escherichia coli*, depresses myocardial responses to endogenous catecholamines [35]. In rat isolated working hearts pretreatment with LPS from *Salmonella typhimurium* induced delayed myocardial protection against ischaemia-reperfusion injury and improved functional recovery [36]. In this study, an enhanced protection occurred when LPS-induced delayed mechanisms were combined with an acute cardioprotective stimulus, such as transient global ischaemia, but as was also pointed out, delayed myocardial adaptation and acute ischaemic preconditioning activated protective mechanisms independently. There have been other studies with *E. coli* LPS, showing that LPS induces delayed protection of the heart against various consequences of acute myocardial ischaemia, including necrotic cell death [37], depressed recovery of contractile function following an ischaemia-reperfusion insult [38, 39] and life-threatening ventricular arrhythmias [37, 40]. Recently it has been demonstrated that the essentially non-toxic derivative of endotoxin, monophosphoryl lipid A (MLA) reduces myocardial ischaemic damage in dogs [41, 42], rabbits [43, 44] and in rats [45] when administered 24 hours prior to ischaemia (see Chapter 9).

In our own experiments, MLA at doses of 10 and 100 µg/kg given to dogs 24 hours before ischaemia, resulted in a dose-dependent reduction in the severity of arrhythmias which occurred during a 25 minute occlusion and then reperfusion of the LAD 24 hours later (Figure 4). For example, the number of VPBs was reduced from 260 ± 77 in the vehicle treated controls to 89 ± 60 with 10 µg/kg MLA, and 28 ± 26 with 100 µg/kg MLA. The incidence of VT was reduced from 63% to 25% with both doses of MLA ($P < 0.05$) and the number of episodes of VT from 12 ± 5 to 1.1 ± 1.1 and 1.6 ± 1.5 ($P < 0.05$), respectively. The incidence of VF in the vehicle controls was 44% during occlusion and 25% of the dogs survived the combined ischaemia-reperfusion insult. MLA significantly reduced the incidence of VF during occlusion (19%, $P < 0.05$) and increased survival to 50% with the higher dose [46].

The mechanisms of the protection induced by LPS and MLA are unclear but there is evidence that either enhanced inducible nitric oxide synthase (NOS) activity [47] or de novo synthesis of myocardial inducible NOS [48] might be involved. This would support the hypothesis of 'cross-tolerance' in that one particular stress triggers protection against the consequences of other types of stress. It seems likely that the same mediator, i.e. enhanced release of NO, plays an important role in the antiarrhythmic effects of both preconditioning and MLA. There is also evidence that in dogs [49] and in rabbits [44] the protective effect of MLA in reducing myocardial ischaemic damage is abolished by the K_{ATP} channel blockers glibenclamide and 5-hydroxydecanoate. However, it is uncertain if the antiarrhythmic effects of MLA involve this channel since it is unlikely to mediate the antiarrhythmic effects of ischaemic preconditioning [50]. It is also of interest that increased activity of 5'-nucleotidase (and the consequent elevation in adenosine levels) is not involved in the mechanism by which preconditioning, or MLA treatment, protects the canine heart against infarction [51, 52].

8. Delayed Protection Against Arrhythmias Induced by Catecholamines

Other, and earlier, examples of pharmacological preconditioning involve the administration of catecholamines. Studies performed in the early 1950s by Rona, Poupa, Selye and Balazs (reviewed in references 34 and 53) showed that the myocardium can be protected against the toxic effects of large doses of isoprenaline by the prior administration of smaller doses of isoprenaline. Historically, these studies almost certainly represent the earliest examples of delayed cardioprotection. These findings are rather suprising, since it is well established that under conditions of ischaemia the release of catecholamines plays a key role in the generation of ventricular arrhythmias. Further, by increasing myocardial contractility, oxygen demand and heat production noradrenaline release contributes to

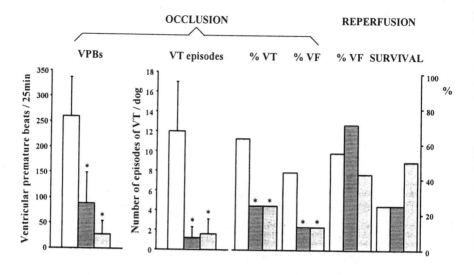

Figure 4. Severity of ventricular arrhythmias during a 25 minute LAD occlusion in anaesthetised dogs (open columns; n = 16) is reduced if the occlusion is preceded by administration of MLA at doses of 10 (hatched columns; n = 8) or 100 µg/kg (filled columns; n =8), 24 hours previously. *P < 0.05 vs. control group

the extent and severity of the myocardial damage that ultimately leads to cell necrosis. One possible explanation why noradrenaline, potentially a substance leading to deleterious effects in the heart, might be protective is that this mediator could mimic the stress situation which occurs when preconditioning is induced by short periods of ischaemia. The administration of noradrenaline may then serve as a preconditioning stimulus but without the harmful consequences of occlusion-induced ischaemia. Exogenous noradrenaline would then represent an example of 'pharmacological preconditioning' (reviewed in reference 54). Indeed, several studies have demonstrated that noradrenaline mimicks the antiarrhythmic effects of classic preconditioning in rat isolated hearts [55] and in anaesthetised dogs in vivo [56]. Recent evidence suggests that pretreatment of rats with noradrenaline in vivo protects against ventricular arrhythmias induced when a coronary artery is occluded 24 hours later [57]. Increasing doses of noradrenaline (1 and 2 µg/kg/minute over a period of 60 minutes), 24 hours before coronary artery occlusion, induced a similar antiarrhythmic protection in anaesthetised dogs (Figure 5). Compared to sham-operated controls (infused with identical volume of saline) there was a significant reduction in the number of VBPs (155 ± 54 vs. 474 ± 169, P < 0.05), episodes of VT (5.1 ± 1.9 vs. 9.4 ± 2.2, P <

0.05) and in the incidence of occlusion-induced VF (11% vs. 63%, P < 0.05) if the dogs had been given noradrenaline 24 hours previously. However, noradrenaline did not increase survival from a combined ischaemia-reperfusion insult (22% vs. 0%, difference not significant).

There are conflicting references in the literature concerning the involvement of catecholamines in the protective effects of preconditioning. In rat isolated hearts, postischaemic recovery of myocardial function is enhanced by a short infusion of isoprenaline given prior to global ischaemia [58, 59]. Also, in some hands the protection induced by preconditioning is abolished by reserpine or by α_1-adrenoceptor blockade [59]. In contrast, in other studies pretreatment with noradrenaline failed to attenuate the severity of ischaemic injury. Further, depletion of endogenous catecholamine stores did not modify the enhanced postischaemic recovery of contractile function associated with preconditioning [60]. Similarly, depletion of catecholamine stores did not influence the antiarrhythmic effect of ischaemic preconditioning in rat isolated hearts [61]. In our canine model of ischaemia-reperfusion the dopamine D_2 receptor agonist Z1046 was profoundly antiarrhythmic [62] suggesting that it is the inhibition of noradrenaline release during ischaemia that is antiarrhythmic. This presynaptic inhibition of endogenous noradrenaline release [63, 64] might also explain the antiarrhythmic effects of exogenously administered noradrenaline.

9. Roles of NO and Bradykinin in Delayed Protection Against Arrhythmias

A number of suggestions have been made to explain the various manifestations of the second window of protection [34, 65]. These include the induction of cytoprotective heat shock proteins [12, 66, 67, 68], the synthesis of a variety of protective enzymes, such as NOS [69, 70, 71] or K^+/Na^+-ATP-ase [34, 57] and increased myocardial anti-oxidant status [72, 73, 74]. There is also some evidence that endogenous myocardial protective substances, such as adenosine are involved as triggers for this protection [75, 76, 77], by activating signal transduction processes, like those involving tyrosine kinase and protein kinase C [78, 79, 80].

It is not known whether cardiac pacing triggers similar mechanisms to those involved in ischaemic preconditioning. However, there is some evidence that endothelium derived mediators are involved in this delayed protection (reviewed recently in references 81 and 82). There are two studies suggesting that mediators similar to those involved in classic ischaemic preconditioning against ventricular arrhythmias play an important role in the delayed antiarrhythmic effects of cardiac pacing. The first is an early study showing that protection at 24 hours was not

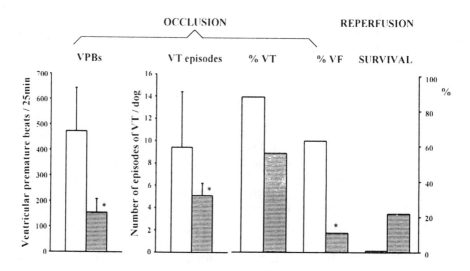

Figure 5. Severity of ventricular arrhythmias during a 25 minute LAD occlusion in control dogs (open columns; n = 8) and in dogs in which increasing doses of noradrenaline (1 and 2 µg/kg/minute) were infused intravenously over a 60 minute period, 24 hours before coronary artery occlusion (hatched columns; n = 9). In dogs given noradrenaline, the number of VPBs, the number of episodes of VT and the incidence of VF during occlusion were significantly reduced. Survival, from combined ischaemia-reperfusion insult, was not significantly increased by noradrenaline. *P < 0.05.

observed if dexamethasone had been administered prior to the pacing stimulus [69]. Thus, in the presence of dexamethasone the incidence of VF was the same in the paced dogs as in the unpaced sham-operated controls (Figure 6). This suggests that NO (or a prostanoid) may be involved, since dexamethasone prevents the induction of enzymes such as NOS and cyclooxygenase II. More recently we have found that aminoguanidine, a more selective inhibitor of inducible NOS [83], when given prior to pacing attenuated the antiarrhythmic effects of cardiac pacing when a coronary artery was occluded 24 hours later [84].

Our hypothesis [2, 26, 81] that NO plays an important role in both the early and delayed phase of protection seems to be confirmed by recent studies from other laboratories. Bolli and colleagues have recently found that NO plays a key role in the delayed protection against myocardial stunning induced by ischaemic stress in rabbits [70]. Similarly Kim and coworkers have demonstrated that, in conscious dogs, brief ischaemic episodes induce delayed enhanced coronary endothelial function in response to endothelium dependent vasodilators, such as bradykinin. This response was associated with an increased production of coronary

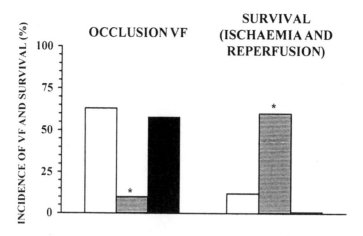

Figure 6. The incidence of VF during coronary occlusion and survival from ischaemia-reperfusion in control dogs (open columns), and dogs subjected to cardiac pacing (four times 5 minutes, at a pacing rate of 220 beats/minute), 24 hours before coronary occlusion, in the absence (hatched columns; n = 10) and in the presence of dexamethasone (filled columns; n = 7). *P < 0.05 vs. control group.

vascular NO metabolites, such as nitrate and nitrite [71]. There is also some experimental evidence that endothelial cell NOS is upregulated by physical exercise [85] resulting in a NO-mediated increase in the calibre of epicardial arteries [86]. This increased vascular NO production following acute exercise also modulates cardiac metabolism [87]. Studies in humans demonstrated that cardiac pacing results in vasodilatation and a reduction in coronary resistance which were abolished after blockade of NO synthesis [88]. Whether the increase in NO production following these various stress stimuli is caused by upregulation of endothelial constitutive NOS or induction of inducible NOS has not been elucidated. It is also not clear what triggers this enhanced production of NO in endothelial cells. We speculate that changes in shear stress resulting from increased coronary blood flow during tachycardia, occurring both during exercise and cardiac pacing, may be involved. It is also not known how long this upregulation or induction lasts after cessation of these stimuli, nor whether such increased NO production is present when endothelial function is compromised as, for example, in atherosclerosis. Some evidence suggests that in a conscious rabbit model, pacing-induced delayed protection was present under even conditions of atherosclerosis although this was not accompanied by an increase in cyclic GMP levels [89].

A further study, which suggests that cardiac pacing-induced delayed protection involves similar mechanisms to that implicated in

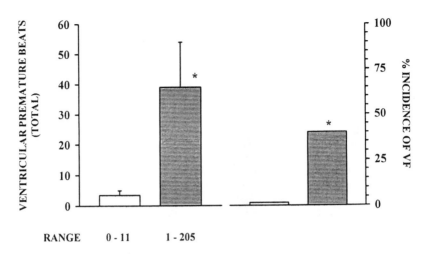

Figure 7. The number of VPBs and the incidence of VF during the pacing procedure in control dogs (paced but not treated; open columns) and in dogs to which icatibant had been given prior to the first episode of pacing (hatched columns). When the preconditioning pacing stimulus was commenced in the presence of icatibant the number of VPBs was markedly increased and 40% of the dogs fibrillated during the pacing procedure. *P < 0.05 vs. control dogs.

classic preconditioning, is that bradykinin, which is both a trigger and mediator of the early antiarrhythmic effects of preconditioning induced both by brief coronary artery occlusions [90] or by cardiac pacing [91], also plays a role in delayed protection [92, 93]. This was examined in dogs in which delayed protection was induced by cardiac pacing in the presence and in the absence of icatibant (Hoe 140), a selective antagonist of bradykinin at bradykinin B_2 receptors. As with the classic preconditioning studies [90, 91], the effects of the preconditioning stimulus itself were more marked in the presence of icatibant. This is illustrated in Figure 7. Thus, only a few VPBs (4 ± 1) occurred in untreated dogs when the pacing was stopped and none of these dogs fibrillated either during or after the pacing procedure. In contrast, when pacing was performed in the presence of icatibant the total number of VPBs was significantly increased (39 ± 2) and 4 out of 10 dogs fibrillated either during the first or the second pacing period.

In those dogs in which icatibant had been given 10 minutes before pacing the protection against the more serious ventricular arrhythmias, such as VF which resulted from coronary artery occlusion 24 hours later, was completely lost. Only 25% of the dogs survived the combined ischaemia-reperfusion insult (Figure 8); this was in contrast to the untreated paced group, in which 63% of the dogs survived. In those dogs in which icatibant was administered after the pacing stimulus but before the occlusion, the protection against arrhythmias was only partially lost. This result indicates that bradykinin, perhaps by releasing NO [26, 93] is both a trigger and a mediator of delayed protection.

10. Conclusion

Although the precise mechanisms of delayed protection are still far from clear there is increasing evidence for the concept that, under normal physiological conditions, coronary vascular endothelial cells generate substances that communicate with cardiac myocytes and help to protect the myocardium against the severe, often fatal, consequences of ischaemia and reperfusion. This is an example of 'cell-to-cell interaction' within the heart and extends the concept that endothelial cells communicate ("talk") to cells concerned with the maintenance of vascular integrity and function by releasing substances with anti-adhesive properties (that protect the endothelial surface against platelet and leucocyte adhesion, e.g. NO, prostacyclin) and that modulate the activity of the underlying vascular smooth muscle by the release of endothelium-derived vasodilators (e.g. prostacyclin, NO) and vasoconstrictors (thromboxane, endothelin).

There are two major consequences of this ability of the coronary vascular endothelium to communicate with cardiac myocytes. The first is to modulate myocardial contractility and metabolism in order to accomodate the myocardium to those conditions which occur during stress, such as during myocardial ischaemia [94]. The second is protection of the potentially ischaemic myocardium by the generation of a variety of 'endogenous protective substances'. The evidence for such diffusible mediators comes from the results of endothelium removal [95] and from the pharmacological manipulation of substances released from endothelial cells (inhibition of synthesis or attenuation of effects at receptor level). There is also some preliminary direct evidence that such substances are generated as a result of brief periods of ischaemia and cardiac pacing and that the levels are higher after a preconditioning stimulus that in its absence [93]. It also seems likely that bradykinin is a key trigger and mediator of this protection, since blockade of bradykinin B_2 receptors with icatibant almost completely abolishes both the early and delayed antiarrhythmic effects of both ischaemic preconditioning and cardiac pacing. The evidence also suggests that much of this protection is mediated by the bradykinin-stimulated generation of NO by endothelium, although there is also some evidence that bradykinin may act as a paracrine mediator in cardiac myocytes by a direct effect on sarcolemmal B_2 receptors. One possible mechanism by which bradykinin could modulate myocardial function is its ability to activate both tyrosine kinases [97] and protein kinase C which translocates from the cytosol to the

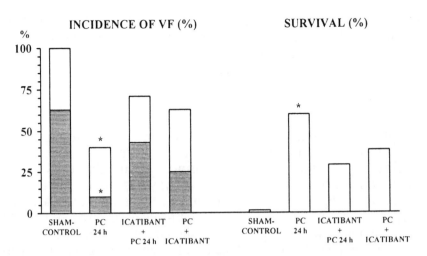

Figure 8. On the left, incidence of VF during occlusion (hatched areas) and reperfusion (open areas); on the right, survival following the combined occlusion-reperfusion insult in control dogs, in paced dogs (PC) and in dogs to which icatibant had been given either before or after cardiac pacing, but prior to coronary occlusion.

membrane, and perhaps to the nucleus [96].

What are the implications of such findings? Presumably, under conditions where endothelial dysfunction is evident, such as hypertension, atherosclerosis and hypercholesterolaemia, the ability to generate such endothelium-derived protective substances may be impaired. This would lead to attenuation of a major pathway for protection within the heart and may explain, at least in part, the increased susceptibility of such patients to the consequences of acute ischaemia, including an increase in arrhythmia severity. Further, drugs that increase the amount of these substances generated by endothelial cells, particularly by inhibiting their breakdown, might be expected to reduce the severity of life-threatening ventricular arrhythmias following coronary artery occlusion. If bradykinin is an important trigger for this cardioprotection then one might expect that arrhythmias to be less severe following administration of angiotensin converting enzyme (ACE) or neutral endopeptidase (NEP) inhibitors. Both families of enzymes are present in cardiac tissue and are involved in catabolism of kinins. Certainly, inhibition of kinin metabolism using NEP inhibitors increases NO production from local coronary microvessels, suggesting that this enzyme plays an important role in kinin-mediated vascular NO production (98). The beneficial cardiac effects of exercise could also be explained by increased endothelial NOS expression leading to increased NO production with resultant modulation of the cAMP/cGMP balance in cardiomyocytes.

It well might be that an approach to the treatment of patients at risk from sudden cardiac death using substances that modulate the heart's own capacity to protect itself against ischaemia might prove a valuable intervention in future clinical practice.

Acknowledgements

Most of our own experiments described and reviewed in this chapter were carried out in the Haemodynamic Laboratory of the Department of Pharmacology at the Albert Szent-Gyorgyi Medical University of Szeged and we wish to thank the the two departmental chairmen involved over this period (1988 to present), Professors Laszlo Szekeres and Julius Gy Papp, for their encouragement and support. We also wish to acknowledge the financial support of the British Council, the European Economic Community (Scientific Network grant No. CIPA CT92 4009), the Hungarian Ministry of Health and Education and the Hungarian National Scientific Committee (OTKA). Among our younger co-workers we particularly appreciate the dedication and enthusiasm of Dr Karoly Kaszala, and of our current PhD students Adrienn Kis, Katalin Gyorgy and Mohamed Ali Rastigar. We are particularly indebted to Erika Toth and Gabor Girst for their valuable technical assistance.

References

1.   Murry CE, Jennings RB, Reimer KA. Preconditioning with ischemia: a delay of lethal cell injury in ischemic myocardium. Circulation 1986; 74: 1124-1136.

2.   Vegh A, Parratt JR. Ischaemic preconditioning markedly reduces the severity of ischaemia and reperfusion-induced arrhythmias; role of endogenous myocardial protective substances. In: Wainwright CL & Parratt JR (eds), Myocardial Preconditioning. Springer, Berlin, 1996: 35-60.

3.   Vegh A, Szekeres L, Udvary E. Effect of blood supply to the normal non-infarcted myocardium on the incidence and severity of early post-occlusion arrhythmias in dogs. Basic Res Cardiol 1987; 82: 159-171.

4.   Vegh A, Komori S, Szekeres L, Parratt JR. Antiarrhythmic effects of preconditioning in anaesthetised dogs and rats. Cardiovasc Res 1992; 26: 487-495.

5.   Russell DC, Lawrie JS, Riemersma RA, Oliver MF. Mechanism of phase 1a and 1b arrhythmia during acute myocardial ischemia in the dog. Am J Cardiol 1984; 53: 307-312.

6.   Kane KA, Parratt JR, Williams FM. An investigation into the characteristics of reperfusion-induced arrhythmias in the anaesthetised rat and their susceptibility to drugs. Br J Pharmacol 1984; 82: 349-357.

7.   Parratt JR, Wainwright CL. Reperfusion arrhythmias - an update. Update in Intensive Care and Emergency Medicine 1988; 5: 293-302.

8.   Haider AW, Tousolio D, Davies GJ. Arrhythmic preconditioning in patients with variant angina. Heart 1996; 75: (Suppl 1), P24 (abstract).

9.   Tamura K, Tsuji H, Nishiue T, Tokunaga S, Iwasaka T. Association of preceding angina with in-hospital life-threatening ventricular tachyarrhythmias and late potentials in patients with a first acute myocardial infarction. Am Heart J 1997; 133: 297-301.

10.   Airaksinen KEJ, Huikuri HV. Antiarrhythmic effect of repeated coronary artery occlusion during balloon angioplasty. J Am Coll Cardiol 1997; 29: 1035-1038.

11.   Kuzuya T, Hoshida S, Yamashita N et al. Delayed effects of sublethal ischemia on the aquisition of tolerance to ischemia. Circ Res 1993; 72: 1293-1299.

12.   Marber MS, Latchman DS, Walker JM, Yellon DM. Cardiac stress protein elevation 24 hours after brief ischemia or heat stress is associated with resistance to myocardial infarction. Circulation 1993; 88: 1264-1272.

13.   Yellon DM, Baxter GF. A "second window of protection" or delayed preconditioning phenomenon: future horizons for myocardial protection? J Mol Cell Cardiol 1995; 27: 1023-1034.

14.   Vegh A, Papp JGy, Kaszala K, Parratt JR. Cardiac pacing in anaesthetised dogs preconditions the heart against arrhythmias when ischaemia is induced 24 h later. J Physiol 1994; 480: 89P (abstract).

15.   Vegh A, Papp JGy, Szekeres L, Kaszala K, Parratt JR. Antiarrhythmic effects of ischaemic preconditioning during the "second window of protection". J Mol Cell Cardiol 1994; 26: A346 (abstract).

16.   Vegh A, Szekeres L, Parratt JR. Transient ischaemia induced by rapid cardiac pacing results in myocardial preconditioning. Cardiovasc Res 1991; 25: 1051-1053.

17.   Kaszala K, Vegh A, Papp JGy, Parratt JR. Time-course of the protection against ischaemia and reperfusion-induced ventricular arrhythmias resulting from brief periods of cardiac pacing. J Mol Cell Cardiol, 1996; 28: 2085-2095.

18.   Szekeres L, Papp JGy, Szilvassy Z, Udvary E, Vegh A. Moderate stress by cardiac pacing may induce both short term and long term cardioprotection. Cardiovasc Res 1993; 27: 593-596.

19.   Sun JZ, Tang XL, Knowlton AA, Park SW, Oiu Y, Bolli R. Late preconditioning against myocardial stunning. An endogenous protective mechanism that confers resistance to postischemic dysfunction 24 h after brief ischemia in conscious pigs. J Clin Invest 1995; 95: 388-403.

20.   Tang XL, Qiu Y, Park SW, Sun JZ, Kalya A, Bolli R. Time course of late preconditioning against myocardial stunning in conscious pigs. Circ Res 1996; 79: 424-434.

21.   Baxter GF, Goma FM, Yellon DM. Duration of the 'second window of protection' following ischaemic preconditioning in the rabbit. J Mol Cell Cardiol 1995; 27: A162 (abstract).

22.   Baxter GF, Goma FM, Yellon DM. Temporal characterisation of the "second window of protection": duration of the anti-infarct effect after ischaemic preconditioning. Circulation 1995; 92 (Suppl I): I- 389 (abstract).

23.   Qiu Y, Tang XL, Park SW, Sun JZ, Kalya A, Bolli R. The early and late phases of ischemic preconditioning. A comparative analysis of their effects on infarct size, myocardial stunning, and arrhythmias in conscious pigs undergoing a 40-minute coronary occlusion. Circ Res 1997; 80: 730-742.

24.   Kis A, Vegh A, Papp JGy, Parratt JR. Repeated pacing widens the time window of delayed protection against ventricular arrhythmias in dogs. J Mol Cell Cardiol 1996; 28: A59 (abstract).

25.   Kis A, Vegh A, Papp JGy, Parratt JR. Repeated pacing markedly prolongs the delayed antiarrhythmic protection in anaesthetised dogs. J Mol Cell Cardiol 1997; 29: A122 (abstract).

26.   Parratt JR, Vegh A. Delayed protection against ventricular arrhythmias by cardiac pacing. Heart 1997; 78: 423-425.

27.   Hull SS, Vanoli E, Adamson PB, Verrier RL, Foreman RD, Schwarz PJ. Exercise training confers anticipatory protection from sudden death during acute myocardial ischemia. Circulation 1994; 89: 548-552.

28.   Zhao G, Zhang X, Xu X, Ochoa M, Hintze TH. Short-term exercise training enhances reflex cholinergic nitric oxide-dependent coronary vasodilation in conscious dogs. Circ Res 1997; 80: 868-876.

29.   Willich SN, Lewis M, Lowel H, Arntz H-R, Schubert F, Schroder R. Physical exertion as a trigger of acute myocardial infarction. N Engl J Med 1993; 329: 1684-1690.

30.   Mittleman MA, Maclure M, Tofler GH, Sherwood JB, Goldberg RJ, Muller JE. Triggering of acute myocardial infarction by heavy physical exertion. Protection against triggering by regular exertion. N Engl J Med 1993; 329: 1667-1683.

31.   Tofler GH, Mittleman MA, Muller JE. Physical activity and the triggering of myocardial infarction: the case for regular exertion. Heart 1996;75: 323-325.

32.   Szekeres L, Szilvassy Z, Udvary E, Vegh A. 7-oxo-PGI$_2$-induced late appearing and long-lasting electrophysiological changes in the heart in situ of the rabbit, guinea pig, dog and cat. J Mol Cell Cardiol 1989; 21: 545-554.

33.   Szekeres L. On the mechanism and possible therapeutic application of delayed cardiac adaptation to stress. Can J Cardiol 1996; 13: 177-185.

34.   Parratt JR, Szekeres L. Delayed protection of the heart against ischaemia. Trends Pharmacol Sci 1995; 16: 351-355.

35.   Parratt JR. Myocardial and circulatory effects of E. coli endotoxin: modification of responses to catecholamines. Br J Pharmacol 1973; 47: 12-25.

36.   Rowland RT, Meng X, Cleveland JC, Meldrum DR, Harken AH, Brown JM. LPS-induced delayed myocardial adaptation enhances acute preconditioning to optimize postischemic cardiac function. Am J Physiol 1997; 272: H2708-H2715.

37.   Wu S, Furman BL, Parratt JR. Delayed protection against ischaemia-induced ventricular arrhythmias and infarct size limitation by the prior administration of Escerichia coli endotoxin. Br J Pharmacol 1996; 118: 2157-2163.

38.   Brown JM, Grosso MA, Terada LS et al. Endotoxin pretreatment increases endogenous myocardial catalase activity and decreases ischemia-reperfusion injury in isolated rat heart. Proc Natl Acad Sci USA 1989; 86: 2526-2530.

39.   McDonough KH, Causey KM. Effects of sepsis on recovery of the heart from 50 min ischemia. Shock 1994; 1: 432-437.

40.   Wu S, Furman BL, Parratt JR. Attenuation by dexamethasone of endotoxin protection against ischaemia-induced ventricular arrhythmias. Br J Pharmacol 1994; 113: 1083-1084.

41.   Yao Z, Rasmussen JL, Hirt JL, Mei DA, Pieper GM, Gross GJ. Effects of monophosphoryl lipid A on myocardial ischemia/reperfusion injury in dogs. J Cardiovasc Pharmacol 1993; 22: 653-663.

42.   Yao Z, Auchampach JA, Pieper GM, Gross GJ. Cardioprotective effects of monophosphoryl lipid A, a novel endotoxin analogue, in the dog. Cardiovasc Res 1993; 27: 832-838.

43.   Baxter GF, Goodwin RW, Wright MJ, Kerac M, Heads RJ, Yellon DM. Myocardial protection after monophosphoryl lipid A: studies of delayed anti-ischaemic properties in rabbit heart. Br J Pharmacol 1996; 117: 1685-1692.

44.   Elliot GT, Comerford ML, Smith JR, Zhao L. Myocardial ischemia/reperfusion protection using monophosphoryl lipid A is abrogated by the ATP-sensitive potassium channel blocker, glibenclamide. Cardiovasc Res 1996; 32: 1071-1080.

45.   Wu S, Furman BL, Parratt JR. Monophosphoryl lipid A reduces arrhythmia severity and infarct size in a rat model of ischaemia. Eur J Pharmacol 1998; 345: 285-287.

46.   Vegh A, Papp JGy, Elliott GT, Parratt JR. Pretreatment with monophosphoryl lipid A (MPL-C) reduces ischaemia-reperfusioninduced arrhythmias in dogs. J Mol Cell Cardiol 1996; 28: A56 (abstract).   .

47.   Zhao L, Weber PA, Smith JR, Comerford ML, Elliott GT. Role of inducible nitric oxide synthase in pharmacological "preconditioning" with monophosphoryl lipid A. J Mol Cell Cardiol 1997; 29: 1567-1576.

48.   Stein B, Frank P, Schmitz W, Scholz H, Thones M. Endotoxin and cytokines induce direct cardioprotective effects in mammalian cardiomyocytes via induction of nitric oxide synthase. J Mol Cell Cardiol 1996; 28: 1631-1639.

49.   Mei DA, Elliott GT, Gross GJ. K_{ATP} channels mediate late preconditioning against infarction produced by monophosphoryl lipid A. Am J Physiol 1996; 271: H2723-H2729.

50.   Vegh A, Papp JGy, Szekeres L, Parratt JR. Are ATP sensitive potassium channels involved in the pronounced antiarrhythmic effects of preconditioning? Cardiovasc Res 1992; 27: 638-543.

51.   Pzyklenk K, Zhao L, Kloner RA, Elliott GT. Cardioprotection with ischemic preconditioning and MLA: role of adenosine-regulating enzymes? Am J Physiol 1996; 271: H1004-H1014.

52.   Przyklenk K, Hata K, Zhao L, Kloner RA, Elliott GT. Disparate effects of preconditioning and MLA on 5'-NT and adenosine levels during coronary occlusion. Am J Physiol 1997; 273: H945-H951.

53.   Vegh A, Parratt JR. Delayed ischaemic peconditioning induced by drugs and by cardiac pacing. In. Wainwright CL, Parratt JR (eds). Myocardial Preconditioning. Springer, Berlin, 1996; 251-260.

54.   Ravingerova T. Mimicking preconditioning with catecholamines. In. Wainwright CL, Parratt JR (eds). Myocardial Preconditioning. Springer, Berlin, 1996; 167-180.

55.   Ravingerova T, Barancik M, Pancza D et al. Contribution to the factors involved in the protective effect of ischemic preconditioning. The role of catecholamines and protein kinase C. Ann NY Acad Sci 1996; 793: 43-54.

56.   Vegh A, Papp JGy, Parratt JR. Intracoronary noradrenaline suppresses ischaemia-induced ventricular arrhythmias in anaesthetised dogs. J Mol Cell Cardiol 1994; 26: LXXXVII (abstract).

57.   Ravingerova T, Song W, Ziegelhoffer A, Parratt J. Delayed antiarrhythmic effect of pretreatment with norepinephrine in rats; the role of Na/KATP-ase. J Mol Cell Cardiol 1995; 27: A162 (abstract).

58.   Locke-Winter CR, Winter CB, Nelson DW, Banerjee A. cAMP stimulation facilitates preconditioning against ischemia-reperfusion through norepinephrine and alpha$_1$ mechanisms. Circulation, 1991; 84: (Suppl 2) II-433 (abstract).

59.   Banerjee A, Locke-Winter C, Rogers KB et al. Preconditioning against myocardial dysfunction after ischemia and reperfusion by an α_1-adrenergic mechanism. Circ Res 1993; 73: 656-670.

60.   Weselcough EO, Baird AJ, Sleph PG, Dzwonzyk S, Murray HN, Grover GJ. Endogenous catecholamines are not necessary for ischaemic preconditioning in the isolated perfused rat heart. Cardiovasc Res 1995; 29: 126-132.

61.   Lawson CS, Hearse DJ. Anti-arrhythmic protection by ischaemic preconditioning in isolated rat hearts is not due to depletion of endogenous catecholamines. Cardiovasc Res 1996; 31: 655-662.

62.   Vegh A, Papp JGy, Semeraro C, Fatehi-Hassanabad Z, Parratt JR. The dopamine receptor agonist Z1046 reduces ischaemia severity in a canine model of coronary artery occlusion. Eur J Pharmacol 1998; 344: 203-213.

63.   Vegh A, Silely M, Papp JGy et al. The dopamine agonist Z1046 suppresses ischaemia-induced ventricular arrhythmias in anaesthetised dogs. J Mol Cell Cardiol 1997; 29: A122 (abstract).

64.   Vegh A, Fatehi-Hassanabad Z, Papp JGy, Semeraro C, Marchini F, Parratt JR. The antiarrhythmic effects of Z1046 are attenuated by domperidone; evidence for the involvement of dopamine DA2 receptors. J Mol Cell Cardiol 1997; 29: A123 (abstract).

65.   Baxter GF, Yellon DM. The "second window of protection" associated with ischaemic preconditioning. In: Marber MS, Yellon DM (eds). Ischaemia, Preconditioning and Adaptation. Oxford: Bios Scientific Publishers, 1996: 113-128.

66.   Currie RW, Karmazyn M, Kloc M, Mailer K. Heat shock response is associated with enhanced post-ischemic ventricular recovery. Circ Res 1988; 63: 543-549.

67.   Yellon DM, Pasini E, Cargnoni A, Marber MS, Latchman DS, Ferrari R. The protective role of heat stress in the ischaemic and reperfused rabbit myocardium. J Mol Cell Cardiol 1992; 24: 895-907.

68.   Nayeem MA, Hess ML, Qian YZ, Loesser KE, Kukreja RC. Delayed preconditioning of cultured adult rat cardiac myocytes: role of 70- and 90-kDa heat stress proteins. Am J Physiol 1997; 273: H861-H868.

69.   Vegh A, Papp JGy, Parratt JR. Prevention by dexamethasone of the marked antiarrhythmic effects of preconditioning induced 20 h after rapid cardiac pacing. Br J Pharmacol 1994; 113: 1081-1082.

70.   Bolli R, Bhatti ZA, Tang X-L, Qiu Y, Zhang Q, Guo Y, Jadoon AK. Evidence that late preconditioning against myocardial stunning in conscious rabbits is triggered by the generation of nitric oxide. Circ Res 1997; 81: 42-52.

71.   Kim SJ, Ghaleh B, Kudej RK, Huang CH, Hintze TH, Vatner SF. Delayed enhanced nitric oxide-mediated coronary vasodilation following brief ischemia and prolonged reperfusion in conscious dogs. Circ Res 1997; 81: 53-59.

72.   Hoshida S, Kuzuya T, Fuji H, Yamashita N, Oe H, Hori M, Suzuki K, Taniguchi N Tada M. Sublethal ischemia alters myocardial antioxidant activity in canine heart. Am J Physiol 1993; 264: H33-H39.

73.   Zhou X, Zhai X, Ashraf M. Direct evidence that initial oxidative stress triggered by preconditioning contributes to second window of protection by endogenous antioxidant enzyme in myocytes. Circulation 1996; 93: 1177--1184.

74.   Baxter GF, Heads RJ, Yellon DM. Oxidative stress and the second window of protection after preconditioning. Circulation 1996; 94: 2992-2993.

75.   Baxter GF, Marber MS, Patel VC, Yellon DM. Adenosine receptor involvement in a delayed phase of myocardial protection 24 hours after ischemic preconditioning. Circulation 1994; 90: 2993-3000.

76.   Baxter GF, Zaman MJS, Kerac M, Yellon DM. Protection against global ischemia in the rabbit isolated heart 24 hours after transient adenosine A_1 receptor activation. Cardiovasc Drugs Ther 1997; 11: 83-85.

77.   Baxter GF, Yellon DM. Time course of delayed myocardial protection after transient adenosine A_1-receptor activation in the rabbit. J Cardiovasc Pharmacol 1997; 29: 631-638.

78.   Imagawa J, Baxter GF, Yellon DM. Genistein, a tyrosine kinase inhibitor, blocks the "second window of protection" 48 h after ischemic preconditioning in the rabbit. J Mol Cell Cardiol 1997; 29: 1885-1893.

79.   Baxter GF, Goma FM, Yellon DM. Involvement of protein kinase C in the delayed cytoprotection following sub-lethal ischaemia in rabbit myocardium. Br J Pharmacol 1995; 115: 222-224.

80.   Fatehi-Hassanabad Z, Parratt JR. Genistein, an inhibitor of tyrosine kinase, prevents the antiarrhythmic effects of preconditioning. Eur J Pharmacol 1998; 338: 67-70.

81.   Parratt JR, Vegh A. Coronary vascular endothelium, preconditioning and arrhythmogenesis. In: Lewis MJ, Shah AM (eds). Endothelial Modulation of Cardiac Function. Reading, Harwood Academic Publishers, 1997; 237-254.

82.   Parratt JR, Vegh A, Kaszala K, Papp JGy. Suppression of life-threatening ventricular arrhythmias by brief periods of ischaemia and by cardiac pacing with particular reference to delayed myocardial protection. In: Marber MS, Yellon DM (eds). Ischaemia, Preconditioning and Adaptation. Oxford: Bios, 1996: 85-111.

83.   Misko TP, Moore WM, Kasten TP, Nichols GA, Corbett JA, Tilton RG, McDaniel ML, Williamson JR, Currie MG. Selective inhibition of the inducible nitric oxide by aminoguanidine. Eur J Pharmacol 1993; 233: 119-125.

84.   Kis A, Vegh A, Papp JGy, Parratt JR. Pacing-induced delayed antiarrhythmic protection is attenuated by aminoguanidine in dogs. J Mol Cell Cardiol 1998; in press.

85.   Sessa WC, Pritchard K, Seyedi N, Wang J, Hintze TH. Chronic exercise in dogs increases coronary vascular nitric oxide production and endothelial cell nitric oxide synthase gene expression. Circ Res 1994; 74: 349-353.

86.   Egashira K, Katsuda Y, Mohri M, Kuga T, Tagawa T, Kubota T, Hirakawa Y, Takeshita A. Role of endothelium-derived nitric oxide in coronary vasodilatation induced by pacing tachycardia in humans. Circ Res 1996; 79: 331-335.

87.   Bernstein RD, Ochoa FY, Xu X, Forfia P, Shen W, Thompson CI, Hintze TH. Function and production of nitric oxide in the coronary circulation of conscious dogs during exercise. Circ Res 1996; 79: 840-848.

88.   Quyyumi AA, Dakak N, Andrews NP, Gillian DM, Panza JA, Canon RO. Contribution of nitric oxide to metabolic coronary vasodilation in the human heart. Circulation 1995; 92: 320-326.

89.   Szekeres L, Szilvassy Z, Ferdinandy P, Nagy I, Karcsu S, Csati S. Delayed cardiac protection against harmful consequences of stress can be induced in experimental atherosclerosis in rabbits. J Mol Cell Cardiol, 1997; 29: 1977-1983.

90.   Vegh A, Papp JGy, Parratt JR. Attenuation of the antiarrhythmic effects of ischaemic preconditioning by blockade of bradykinin B_2 receptors. Br J Pharmacol 1994; 113: 1167-1172.

91.   Kaszala K, Vegh A, Papp JGy, Parratt JR. Modification by bradykinin B_2 receptor blockade of protection by pacing against ischaemia-induced arrhythmias. Eur J Pharmacol 1997; 308: 51-60.

92.   Vegh A, Kaszala K, Papp JGy, Parratt JR. Delayed myocardial protection by pacing-induced preconditioning: a possible role for bradykinin. Br J Pharmacol 1995; 116: 288P (abstract).

93.   Parratt JR, Vegh A, Zeitlin J et al. Bradykinin and endothelial-cardiac myocyte interactions in ischemic preconditioning. Am J Cardiol 1997; 80 (3A): 124A-131A.

94.   Lewis M, Shah A (eds). Endothelial Modulation of Cardiac Function. Reading: Harwood Academic Publishers. 1997.

95.   Fatehi-Hassanabad Z, Furman BL, Parratt JR. Endothelium and ischaemic preconditioning in rat isolated perfused hearts. J Physiol 1996; 494: 112P-113P (abstract).

96.   Wilson S, Song W, Kaszala K et al. Delayed cardioprotection is associated with the subcellular relocalisation of ventricular protein kinase C, but not p42/44MAPK. Mol Cell Biochem 1996; 160/161: 225-230.

97.   Fleming I, Fisslthaler B, Busse R. Calcium signalling in endothelial cells involve activation of tyrosine kinases and leads to activation of mitogen-activated protein kinases. Circ Res 1995; 76: 522-529.

98.   Zhang X, Xu X, Fortia PR, Nasiletti A, Hintze TH. Neutral endopeptidase (NEP) and angiotensin converting enzyme (ACE) modulate nitric oxide (NO) via local kinin formation production from canine coronary microvessels. Circulation 1996; 94: (suppl), 349.

5

Intracellular Signalling Mechanisms in Myocardial Adaptation to Ischaemia

D K Das

1. Introduction

Living organisms exhibit specific responses when confronted with sudden environmental changes. The ability of cells to acclimatise to a new environment is the basis of adaptive modification. Adaptation involves a number of cellular and biochemical alterations including (i) changes in metabolic homeostasis and (ii) reprogramming of gene expression. Changes in metabolic pathways are generally short-lived and reversible; the consequences of reprogrammed gene expression are long-term and may lead to permanent alteration.

The heart possesses a remarkable ability to adapt to many stressful situations. Tissue stress is a component of many heart diseases including atherosclerosis, vascular spasm, thrombosis, cardiomyopathy, and congestive heart failure. The idea that excessive stress can play a key role in the pathogenesis of ischaemic heart disease suggests that designing methods for the prevention of stress-induced myocardial injury might be an important approach to the prevention and treatment of these diseases. Indeed, creating a stress response by repeated ischaemia and reperfusion or subjecting the heart to heat or oxidative stress can equip it to withstand further stress. Repeated stress exposure adapts the heart to withstand more severe stress probably by upregulating cellular defences and direct accumulation of intracellular mediators. Thus, the powerful cardioprotective effect of adaptation is likely to originate at the cellular and molecular levels. This chapter will focus specifically on the molecular signalling pathways that are known to be involved in myocardial adaptation to ischaemia.

2. Stress Adaptation in the Heart

Classic ischaemic preconditioning is the earliest stress response that occurs during repeated episodes of brief ischaemia and reperfusion, and can render the myocardium more tolerant to a subsequent potential lethal ischaemic injury [1, 2]. Ischaemic adaptation occurs in two different steps: (i) an early or immediate effect (classic ischaemic preconditioning); and (ii) a late effect (delayed adaptation or second window of protection) which may occur after approximately 24 hours and may last up to several days. The early transient response has been shown to be associated with decreased reperfusion-induced arrhythmias, increased recovery of postischaemic contractile function, and reduction of infarct size (see references 3 and 4 for review). The delayed adaptive protection is thought to be mediated by gene expression, transcriptional regulation and subsequent protein synthesis [5, 6]. These genes include those encoding for proto-oncogenes (c-fos, c-myc, and c-jun); the heat shock proteins (HSP's), HSP27, HSP60, HSP70, and HSP89 (see Chapter 7); and antioxidants such as manganese superoxide dismutase (see Chapter 8), catalase, heme oxygenase and several others [7-12] (see also Chapter 6). A number of factors which were found to regulate classic ischaemic preconditioning (early adaptation), have also been found to play a crucial role in the delayed adaptation to ischaemia. For example, three principal players in classic ischaemic preconditioning, adenosine, ATP-sensitive potassium channels (K_{ATP}), and protein kinase C (PKC), are critically involved in the second window of protection [13, 14].

3. Signal Transduction Pathways in Adaptation

Protein phosphorylation is central to a wide variety of cellular processes that control signal transduction. Protein phosphorylation is a rapidly reversible process which regulates intracellular signalling in response to a specific stress [15]. Protein phosphorylation is mediated by a number of protein kinases that can be grouped into two major classes:

(i) kinases which phosphorylate proteins on their tyrosine residues, i.e. tyrosine kinases.
(ii) kinases which phosphorylate serine/threonine residues, e.g. protein kinase A (PKA), PKC, and casein kinases.

4. Protein Tyrosine Kinase Signalling

Tyrosine kinases can activate a number of different intracellular signalling pathways including tyrosine phosphorylation in case of phospholipase C-γ (PLCγ) and phospholipase D (PLD) [16], conformational changes induced by binding of the SH2 domain to phosphotyrosine for phosphoinositol-3-hydroxy (PI3) kinases [17] as well as translocation to the plasma membrane for stimulation of Ras guanine nucleotide exchange by Sos [18].

Our laboratory has demonstrated that brief ischaemia and reperfusion triggers a signalling pathway by potentiating tyrosine kinase phosphorylation [19, 20]. The signal transduction involves PLD which subsequently transmits the signal via the activation of mitogen activated protein (MAP) kinases. Our results clearly indicated a role of tyrosine kinase, because inhibition of tyrosine kinase phosphorylation by genistein almost completely blocked the activation of PKC, MAP kinases and MAPKAP kinase 2. Subsequently, we were able to identify p38 MAP kinase as one of the potential targets for tyrosine kinase phosphorylation [21] (see below).

5. Phospholipase D Signalling

Phospholipid turnover plays a crucial role in intracellular signalling processes. At least three phospholipases are known to be regulated by the receptor protein tyrosine kinases, phospholipase A2, PLCγ and PLD. The primary step of the signal transduction pathway for the activation of PKC involves the stimulation of PLC, generating the second messenger diacylglycerol [22]. Several studies demonstrated that activation of PLD plays a crucial role in ischaemic preconditioning [23, 24]. PLD preferentially acts on phosphatidylcholine generating phosphatidic acid which is readily metabolised by a phosphohydrolase present in the heart into diacylglycerol. Activation of PLD was documented in the ischaemic and reperfused [24] as well as in preconditioned hearts [23, 25]. Activators of PLD simulated the effects of ischaemic preconditioning while the inhibition of PLD blocked the beneficial (antiarrhythmic) effects of preconditioning. Using specific polyclonal antibodies to PLD, we directly inhibited the phospholipase, and simultaneously reduced the amount of diacylglycerol and phosphatidic acid as well as significantly inhibiting the stimulation of PKC [26]. In addition, this anti-PLD antibody blocked the beneficial effects of ischaemic preconditioning, evidenced by the increased incidence of ventricular arrhythmias. In a previous study, we found that the same anti-PLD antibody blocked ischaemia-reperfusion-mediated activation of PLD [24]. PLD catalyses the hydrolysis of the terminal diester bond of phosphatidylcholine with the formation of choline and phosphatidic acid, the latter of which serves as a substrate for diacylglycerol biosynthesis by the action of phosphatidic acid phosphohydrolase. Diacylglycerol may serve as a second messenger leading to the activation of PKC. PLD also catalyses a transphosphatidylation reaction in which the phosphatidyl moiety of the phospholipid is transferred to a nucleophilic alcohol producing a corresponding phosphatidyl alcohol [27]. Ischaemia-reperfusion was shown to activate PLD, generating intracellular phosphatidic acid, part of which is converted to diacylglycerol [24]. Additionally, activation of myocardial PLD by sodium oleate resulted in a significant improvement of post-ischaemic functional recovery and attenuation of cellular injury suggesting that PLD signalling in the ischaemic myocardium is beneficial for recovery of the heart.

In addition to PLD, other phospholipases including PLA_2 and PLC also become activated in response to ischaemia and reperfusion [22]. However, activation of PLA_2 causes the generation of arachidonic acid and lysophosphoglycerides which are detrimental to the heart [28]. Activation of PLC also generates diacylglycerol, but it causes the production of inositol triphosphate which mobilises Ca^{2+} from the intracellular compartments [29]. Thus, unlike the detrimental effects of PLA_2 and PLC, activation of PLD is beneficial to the heart. As we have seen, activation of PLD produces phosphatidic acid while activation of PLC produces diacylglycerol. However, these two products of hydrolysis are easily convertible, catalysed by two enzymes, diacylglycerol kinase and phosphatidic acid phosphohydrolase. Inhibition of diacylglycerol kinase does not affect the amount of diacylglycerol or phosphatidic acid generated during ischaemia-reperfusion. On the contrary, phosphatidic acid phosphohydrolase inhibition leads to an enhancement of phosphatidic acid in concert with a reduction in diacylglycerol [22], suggesting that PLD activity is solely responsible for the generation of phosphatidic acid. Additionally, it indirectly contributes to diacylglycerol generation since part of the phosphatidic acid is hydrolysed to diacylglycerol by phosphatidic acid phosphohydrolase [30]. In fact, PLD-mediated stimulus-response couplings are known to exist in several cell types.

Signal transduction mediated by growth factors such as epidermal growth factor, platelet-derived growth factor and insulin occurs through protein tyrosine kinase found on the plasma membrane [31]. The earliest events for such signal transduction include activation of $PLC\gamma$ and PLD [32, 33]. Several agonists can also enhance PLD activation through protein tyrosine phosphorylation. For example, in human embryonic kidney cells, expression of the M_3 muscarinic receptor increased tyrosine phosphorylation of various cellular proteins and PLD in response to carbachol [34]. The involvement of protein tyrosine phosphorylation in PLD activation was supported from the observations that tyrosine kinase inhibitors such as genistein and tyrphostin blocked PLD activation [35] and, conversely, that PLD activation was increased upon treatment with the tyrosine phosphatase inhibitors vanadate and pervanadate [36]. Many oxidants such as H_2O_2 can increase protein tyrosine phosphorylation [37] in conjunction with PLD activation [38]. In neutrophils and HL-60 cells, oxygen free

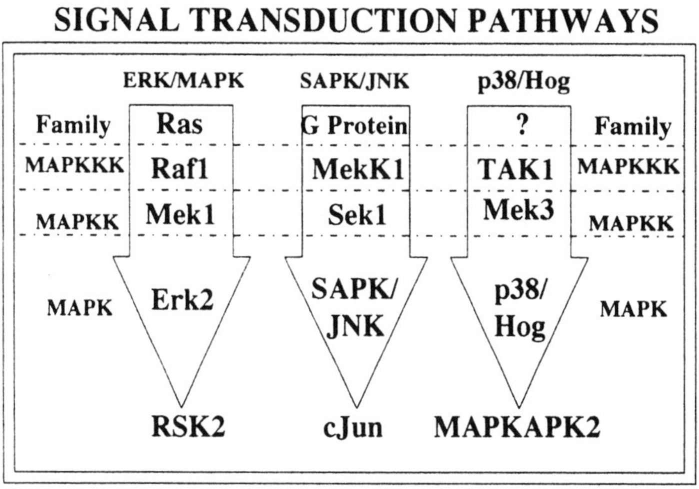

SIGNAL TRANSDUCTION PATHWAYS

	ERK/MAPK	SAPK/JNK	p38/Hog	
Family	Ras	G Protein	?	Family
MAPKKK	Raf1	MekK1	TAK1	MAPKKK
MAPKK	Mek1	Sek1	Mek3	MAPKK
MAPK	Erk2	SAPK/JNK	p38/Hog	MAPK
	RSK2	cJun	MAPKAPK2	

Figure 1. Mitogen activated protein kinases (MAPKs) are classified in three major families: the ERKs (classic MAPK); SAPK/JNK; and p38 kinase. MAPKs are activated in a cascade or relay fashion. The immediately upstream kinases are MAPK kinases (MAPKK; Mek 1, Sek 1 and Mek 3 in this schema). MAPKKs are activated by MAPKK kinases (MAPKKK; Raf 1. MekK 1 and TAK 1 in this schema). For more detail, see text below.

radicals generated by f-Met-Leu-Phe resulted in increased protein tyrosine phosphorylation and PLD activation [39]. Genistein not only blocked the oxidant-mediated protein tyrosine phosphorylation in endothelial cells, but also a correlation between tyrosine kinase inhibition and PLD activation was observed with genistein [40].

Although evidence supports a role of tyrosine kinases in PLD activation, the mechanisms of activation remain unknown. It is possible that PLD activation is the direct manifestation of protein tyrosine kinase phosphorylation. It is also possible that tyrosine kinase generates other intermediate proteins which are instrumental for PLD activation. A number of recent studies have identified MAP kinases as targets for tyrosine phosphorylation as described earlier. In a recent study, ischemic preconditioning-mediated activation of PLD was found to be inhibited by a tyrosine kinase blocker, genistein while the preconditioning effect was almost abolished by the genistein treatment [19]. Additionally, preconditioning rat hearts stimulated multiple protein kinases including PKC, MAP kinase, and MAPKAP kinase 2 which were inhibited by genistein, suggesting the existence of a tyrosine kinase coupled PLD pathway for ischaemic preconditioning and implicating the involvement of multiple protein kinases in myocardial adaptation to ischaemia.

6. Protein Kinase C Signalling

A role of PKC in ischaemic preconditioning has been widely investigated. Short term ischaemia as well as ischaemia followed by reperfusion were previously shown to translocate and activate PKC [41]. Furthermore, both α_1 receptor stimulation and Ca^{2+} can translocate and activate PKC [42, 43]. Given the fact that both α_1-receptor activation and intracellular Ca^{2+} overloading occur during ischaemia-reperfusion, it was not surprising when ischaemic preconditioning, consisting of repeated ischaemia and reperfusion, was also found to translocate and activate PKC [44, 45]. Interestingly, it has long been known that PKC can activate gene transcription [46]. Indeed, many genes were found to be activated in the preconditioned myocardium [5, 9-12, 47-50]. Thus, PKC which is activated by endogenous compounds (namely catecholamines, adenosine, diacylglycerol) may be instrumental for gene expression leading to the translation into proteins.

As mentioned earlier, it has been demonstrated that PKC activation is an important step in the mechanism of adaptive protection of the heart [30, 31, 51]. The PKC hypothesis received further support from the observations that any agent that can activate PKC can also precondition the heart. For example, α_1, angiotensin AT_1 and bradykinin B_2 receptor agonists can activate PKC [52]. Phenylephrine, angiotensin and bradykinin have been shown to precondition the hearts when infused prior to ischaemia [53, 54].

A variety of stress signals have been found to translocate and activate PKC. For example, mechanical stress induced by stretching can activate PKC in cultured myocytes [55]. Immediately after stretching, activation of phosphatidyl inositol turnover was observed suggesting a role of PLC in PKC activation. Our laboratory demonstrated that even short-term ischaemia or ischaemia followed by reperfusion could translocate and activate PKC [41] and demonstrated a role of PKC in ischaemic preconditioning [30] supporting the findings from other laboratories.

7. Mitogen Activated Protein Kinases

Three distinct mammalian MAP kinases, each with apparently unique signalling pathways, have been identified (Figure 1):

(i) the ERK group, the originally-defined MAP kinases, also called
    p42/p44 MAP kinases;
(ii) the p38 MAP kinase;

(iii) the stress activated protein (SAP) kinase group (also known as c-
      jun-N-terminal kinase or SAPK/JNK);

In mammalian cells, mitogenic signals are transmitted from the
cytoplasm into the nucleus by the nuclear translocation of p42/p44 MAP
kinase isoforms (extracellular signal regulated kinases, ERK1 and
ERK2) [56]. Although the kinase cascades have been well characterised
for prokaryotic systems, their precise roles and mechanisms of
activation in mammalian systems are far from clear. MAP kinase signal
transduction pathways are likely to involve activation of Ras or Raf-1
which in turn induces MAP kinase kinase (MAPKK or MKK) and MAP
kinases. It is also known that Raf-1 kinases possess MAPKKK activity
and lie upstream from MKKs and MAP kinases in various cell types
[57]. A recent study has demonstrated that hypoxia and
hypoxia/reoxygenation activated raf-1, MKK and MAP kinases in
cultured rat cardiomyocytes. Raf-1 operates downstream cell surface-
associated tyrosine kinases and upstream from MAP kinases. Raf is not
strictly a member of the MEKK family, but it is a functional analogue.
Ras is part of the signal transduction chain extending from extracellular
signals to transcriptional regulation in the nucleus. Upon activation,
tyrosine kinase recruits a number of proteins including Ras-specific
guanine nucleotide releasing proteins which then regulate the binding of
Ras with GTP, thereby potentiating the Ras signal. Ras proteins then
interact with Raf kinases to induce downstream signals activating MAP
kinases and other protein kinases. Once Raf is activated, then Ras is no
longer required. The precise mechanism by which Ras controls Raf-1 is
poorly understood. The binding of Raf-1 to Ras is largely GTP
dependent and requires the effector region of Ras and the regulatory
region of Raf-1.

8. p38 MAP Kinase Signalling

Both oxidative stress and heat stress rapidly activate p38 MAP kinase
and MAPKAP kinase 2 leading to the phosphorylation of HSP27 [58].
To further define the role of p38/MAPKAP kinase 2 signalling in
ischaemia-reperfusion, we used a specific blocker of p38 MAP kinase,
SB203580, prior to ischaemia and reperfusion. The results of our study
demonstrated that ischaemia-reperfusion resulted in the translocation of
p38 MAP kinase into the cytoplasm. The beneficial effects of
myocardial adaptation to stress by repeated ischaemia and reperfusion
were abolished by blocking p38 MAP kinase with SB203580, with
simultaneous inhibition of MAPKAP kinase 2, suggesting a role of the
p38 MAPkinase-MAPKAP kinase 2 signalling pathway [59]. Activation
of p38 MAP kinase with anisomycin mimicked ischaemic
preconditioning (Figure 2).

Unlike p42/p44 MAP kinases (ERKs), which are readily activated by growth signals via a Ras-dependent signal transduction pathway [60], the activation of SAPK/JNK and p38 MAP kinase is potentiated by diverse stresses and pro-inflammatory cytokines [61]. However, the SAPK/JNK and p38 MAP kinase cascades appear to be involved in distinct cellular functions because they possess different cellular targets and locate on different signalling pathways. For example, JNK activates c-Jun while p38 MAP kinase stimulates MAPKAP kinase2 [62, 63], which in turn leads to the phosphorylation of HSP27 [64]. The precise mechanism of p38 MAP kinase activation is not known, but its activation appears to be regulated by dual phosphorylation on Thr and Tyr within the motif Thr-Gly-Tyr [65]. Recently, the nucleus has been shown to be a target for the p38 MAP kinase signal transduction [66].

Although the activation of p38 MAP kinase requires dual phosphorylation like other members of MAP kinases family, the substrate specificity of p38 MAP kinase is quite different from that of SAPK/JNK or ERK subgroups of MAP kinases. Thus, unlike other MAP kinases, p38 MAP kinase activates MAPKAP kinase 2. It is speculated that p38 MAP kinase signalling has a distinct function in the cell, and this was supported by the recent findings that pro-inflammatory cytokines cause the activation of p38 MAP kinase which in turn results in the phosphorylation of HSP27 [67, 68]. Recently, two MAP kinase kinases (MKK3 and MKK4) have been discovered, the former being specific for p38 MAP kinase, while the latter can activate both p38 MAP kinase and SAPK/JNK [69] suggesting that p38 and SAPK/JNK may sit at the crossroads of the stress-activated signal transduction pathway.

9. MAPKAP Kinase 2

p38 MAP kinase [70] has a very specific cellular target, MAPKAP kinase 2 [71]. The results of a number of recent studies from our laboratory now suggest that PKC may not be the ultimate link between ischaemic preconditioning and myocardial adaptation. These include the abundance of MAP kinase-activated protein, kinase MAPKAP kinase 2, in heart, rapid activation of MAPKAP kinase 2 by stresses including heat stress, oxidative stress and ischaemia-reperfusion, and most importantly, it is MAPKAP kinase 2, and not PKC that can phosphorylate the small heat shock proteins, HSP25/HSP27, which are also activated by ischaemic preconditioning. MAPKAP kinase 2 is regulated by tyrosine kinase because, inhibition of tyrosine kinase abolished preconditioning-mediated activation of PKC, MAP kinase and MAPKAP kinase 2 [19]. First isolated as an in vitro substrate for ERKs, MAPKAP kinase 2, a Ser/Thr kinase, has been shown to be phosphorylated and activated by MAP kinases both in vivo and in vitro.

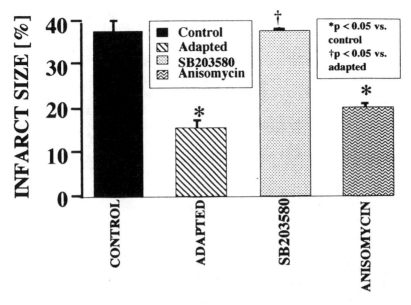

Figure 2. Involvement of p38 MAP kinase in ischaemic preconditioning was demonstrated in rat heart. Preconditioning resulted in significant limitation of infarct size (adapted). Pretreatment with the selective inhibitor of p38 MAP kinase, SB203580, resulted in loss of protection. Conversely, treatment with anisomycin, an activator of both p38 MAP kinase and SAPK/JNK, resulted in protection comparable to that seen with preconditioning.

MAPKAP kinase 2 is a 370-amino acid protein containing a highly conserved catalytic domain of proline-rich N-terminus and a C-terminus region containing a MAP kinase phosphorylation site at Thr-334. The physiological functions of MAPKAP kinase 2 remain unknown. This kinase is largely expressed in myocardium and skeletal muscle [58]. A number of recent studies suggested that MAPKAP kinase 2 may play a significant role in the stress-activated signal transduction potentiated by diverse environmental stresses, pro-inflammatory cytokines as well as a variety of mitogens [71]. In addition, phorbol ester, heat shock and oxidative stress can also activate MAPKAP kinase 2 in cardiac myoblast cells [58]. MAPKAP kinase 2 is a down-stream protein kinase in the stress-activated signal transduction pathway. Northern blot analysis indicated that this enzyme is highly expressed in heart tissues [58] suggesting that MAPKAP kinase 2 may function in myocardium in response to stress or mitogenic stimulation. In addition, MAPKAP kinase 2 activity in cardiomyocytes is stimulated by a myocardial hypertrophic factor (unpublished observation), by oxidative stress and by heat shock. Recombinant MAPKAP kinase 2 phosphorylates HSP27 in cardiomyocytes, determined by in vitro phosphorylation assay. The known association between MAPKAP kinase 2 and the HSPs gives rise to the possibility that the kinase may be involved in a stress-related response of myocardium which leads to cardioprotection. Our previous studies indicated that stresses including heat shock, oxidative stress and phorbol ester treatment of cultured cardiac myoblast cells resulted in a rapid increase in cellular MAPKAP kinase 2 activity [58].

In a recent study, we observed that the enzymatic activity of MAPKAP kinase 2 (determined by in vitro kinase assay using MBP as a substrate) resulted from the activation of the tissue ERK and/or p38 MAP kinases. In in vitro studies, both ERK and p38 MAP kinases can phosphorylate and activate MAPKAP kinase 2 [72, 73]. To detect tissue/cellular MAPKAP kinase 2 activity, the synthetic peptide derived from N-terminus of glycogen synthase is widely used as a specific substrate. In our study, 20 mM H-7 was utilised in the kinase assay to inhibit enzyme activities mediated through other cellular kinases, including cAMP-dependent protein kinase (Ki = 3.0 mM), PKC (Ki = 6.0 mM), and protein kinase G (Ki = 5.8 mM). The specificity of the kinase assay using whole tissue lysate and the peptide substrate has already been demonstrated from the observations that induced MAPKAP kinase 2 activity (detected using an in vitro kinase assay with whole tissue lysates and synthetic peptide as substrate) was inhibited in the presence of the competitive inhibitory peptide for MAPKAP kinase 2 [74]. The MAP kinase activity thus truly reflects the total MAP kinase activity, including ERKs, SAPK/JNK or p38 MAP kinases.

10. Gene Expression

Studies from different laboratories have demonstrated that ischaemic preconditioning results in the induction of the expression of large variety of stress-induced genes [16, 27-30, 75-78] (see chapter 6). Using subtractive hybridisation and differential display techniques, our laboratory demonstrated that preconditiong can also induce a number of mitochondrial genes as well as the fatty acid transport (FAT) gene [5, 9-12].

HSP27 is an early target of phosphorylation upon stimulation by serum or a variety of mitogens, cytokines, inducers of differentiation and a variety of stress conditions [75]. As mentioned earlier, a previous study from our laboratory demonstrated the induction of HSP27 in rat hearts after ischaemic preconditioning. Phosphorylation regulates HSP27 function which may provide cardioprotection during myocardial ischaemia and reperfusion. It has been demonstrated that HSP27 phosphorylation is regulated by the activation of MAPKAP kinase 2, as described above [74].

The precise physiological role of MAPKAP kinase 2 in the regulation of HSP expression is not known, but this kinase has been

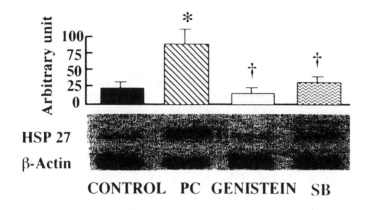

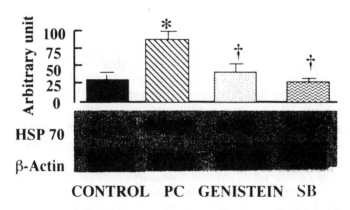

Figure 3. Northern blots showing the effects of preconditioning (PC) on the induction of HSP27 and HSP70 mRNAs in rat heart. PC resulted in significant induction of mRNA for each HSP. Pretreatment with either genistein, a tyrosine kinase inhibitor, or SB203580 (SB) resulted in almost complete abolition of induction. * P < 0.05 compared with control; † P < 0.05 compared with PC.

implicated as a down-stream mediator of the p38 MAP kinase cascade. It has been shown that, except for MAPKAP kinase 2, no other kinases, including PKC, are capable of inducing phosphorylation of HSP27 directly. Induction of the expression of HSP27 in response to diverse stresses has been demonstrated. For example, both ischaemia-reperfusion and oxidative stress can induce the expression of HSP27 in mammalian hearts [6, 7, 76, 77]. The fact that phosphorylation of HSP27 precedes its activation [78], and that HSP27 is induced in response to stress including ischaemic preconditioning, suggests a role of HSP27 in ischaemic preconditioning and myocardial adaptation.

Preconditioning-mediated HSP induction is inhibited by blocking tyrosine phosphorylation or p38 MAP kinase activation [79]

(Figure 3). Results of the Northern analysis are shown in Figure 3. Preconditioning resulted in a significant enhancement of induction of HSP27 and HSP70 expression: for HSP27, the induction was 3.2-fold increased while 3.5-fold induction was noticed for HSP70. Both genistein and SB203580 completely abolished the induction of the expression of these HSPs suggesting that such induction is achieved through a tyrosine kinase/p38 MAP kinase signal transduction pathway.

11. Conclusion

In summary, stress induced by single or multiple brief periods of ischaemia and reperfusion renders the heart more tolerant to subsequent lethal ischaemic insult. This phenomenon has been termed ischaemic preconditioning and produces both a short-term protection and a "second window of protection". The latter is a long-term adaptive process mediated by gene expression and transcriptional regulation. The initial ischaemic-stress signal is likely to be triggered by the activation of protein tyrosine kinases which then transmit the signal by activating PLD, then through the MAP kinases and onto MAPKAP kinase 2 in a relay-type fashion.

Constitutive cellular protection against acute stress such as ischaemia is provided by a variety of intracellular components including antioxidants and HSPs. These components are an integral part of the defence system of the heart. When myocardial cells sense stress, they readily react by augmenting these elements of the defence system. Many stress-regulated proteins are likely to comprise the defence system because, they undergo rapid changes as a consequence of the development of stress associated with a large number of pathological states, including ischaemia and reperfusion. The intracellular signal transduction is mediated by the action of multiple kinases, and is likely to be instrumental for the induction of mRNAs for a variety of inducible stress proteins involved in cellular protection or repair of injury. This adaptive defence phenomenon related to specific gene expression may represent the ultimate adaptive stress response in the myocardium.

Acknowledgements

This study was supported in part by NIH grants HL 22559 and HL 33889.

References

1.   Murry CE, Jennings RB, Reimer KA. Preconditioning with ischemia: a delay of lethal cell injury in ischemic myocardium. Circulation 1986; 74: 1124-1136.

2.   Flack J, Kimura Y, Engelman RM, Das DK. Preconditioning the heart by repeated stunning improves myocardial salvage. Circulation 1991; 84: III369-III374.

3.   Yellon DM, Baxter GF, Garcia-Dorado D, Heusch G, Sumeray MS. Ischaemic preconditioning: present position and future directions. Cardiovasc Res 1998; 37: 21-33.

4.   Parratt JR. Protection of the heart by ischaemic preconditioning: mechanisms and possibilities for pharmacological exploitation. Trends Pharmacol Sci 1994; 15: 19-25.

5.   Maulik N, Das DK. Hunting for differentially expressed mRNA species in preconditioned myocardium. Ann N Y Acad Sci 1996; 793: 240-258.

6.   Das DK, Moraru II, Maulik N, Engelman RM. Gene expression during myocardial adaptation to ischemia and reperfusion. Ann N Y Acad Sci 1994; 723: 292-307.

7.   Das DK, Engelman RM, Kimura Y. Molecular adaptation of cellular defenses following preconditioning of the heart by repeated ischemia. Cardiovasc Res 1993; 27: 578-584.

8.   Yamashita N, Hoshida S, Nishida M et al. Time course of tolerance to ischemia-reperfusion injury and induction of heat shock protein 72 by heat stress in the rat heart. J. Mol Cell Cardiol 1997; 29: 1815-1821.

9.   Maulik N, Sharma HS, Das DK. Induction of the haem oxygenase gene expression during the reperfusion of ischemic rat myocardium. J Mol Cell Cardiol 1996; 28: 1261-1270.

10.   Moraru II, Engelman DT, Engelman RM et al. Myocardial ischemia triggers rapid expression of mitochondrial genes. Surg Forum 1994; 45: 315-317.

11.   Sharma HS, Maulik N, Gho BCG, Das DK, Verdouw PD. Coordinated expression of heme oxygenase-1 and ubiquitin in the porcine heart subjected to ischemia and reperfusion. Mol Cell Biochem 1996; 157: 111-116.

12.   Maulik N, Das DK. Molecular cloning, sequencing and expression analysis of a fatty acid transport gene in rat heart induced by ischemic preconditioning and oxidative stress. Mol Cell Biochem 1996; 160/161: 241-247.

13.   Baxter GF, Marber MS, Patel VC, Yellon DM. Adenosine receptor involvement in a delayed phase of myocardial protection 24 hours after ischemic preconditioning. Circulation 1994; 90: 2993-3000.

14.   Baxter GF, Goma FFM, Yellon DM. Involvement of protein kinase C in the delayed cytoprotection following sublethal ischemia in rabbit myocardium. Br J Pharmacol 1995; 115: 222-224.

15.   Hunter T, Alexander CB, Cooper JA. Protein tyrosine kinases. Ann Rev Biochem 1995; 54: 897-930.

16.   Sadowski HB, Shuai K, Darnell JE, Gilman MZ. A common nuclear signal transduction pathway activated by growth factor and cytokine receptors. Science 1993; 261: 1739-1744.

17.   Carpenter CL, Auger KR, Chanudhuri M et al. Phosphoinositide 3-kinase is activated by phosphopeptides that bind to the SH2 domains of the 85-kDa subunit. J Biol Chem 1993; 268: 9478-9483.

18.   Quilliam LA, Huff SY, Rabun KM et al. Membrane-targeting potentiates guanine nucleotide exchange factor CDC25 and SOS1 activation of Ras transforming activity. Proc Natl Acad Sci USA 1994; 91: 8512-8516.

19.   Maulik N, Watanabe M, Zu YL et al. Ischemic precon-ditioning triggers the activation of MAP kinases and MAPKAP kinase 2 in rat hearts. FEBS Lett 1996; 396: 233-237.

20.   Das DK, Maulik N, Yoshida T, Engelman RM, Zu YL. Preconditioning potentiates molecular signaling for myocardial adaptation to ischemia. Ann N Y Acad Sci 1996; 793: 191-209.

21.   Maulik N, Watanabe M, Tosaki A et al. Tyrosine kinase regulation of phospholipase D-protein C kinase pathway in ischemic preconditioning. J Am Coll Cardiol 1996; 27: 385A (abstract).

22.   Prasad MR, Popescu L, Moraru II, Liu X, Engelman RM, Das DK.Role of phospholipase A2 and phospholipase C in myocardial ischemic reperfusion injury. Am J Physiol 1991; 260: H877-H883.

23.   Cohen MV, Liu Y, Liu GS et al. Phospholipase D plays a major role in ischemic preconditioning in rabbit heart. Circulation 1996; 94: 1713-1718.

24.   Moraru II, Popescu L, Maulik N, Liu X, Das DK. Phospholipase D signaling in ischemic heart. Biochim Biophys Acta 1992; 1139: 148-154.

25.   Trifan OC, Popescu LM, Tosaki A, Cordis G, Das DK. Ischemic preconditioning involves phospho-lipase D. Annals N.Y. Acad Sci 1996; 793: 485-488.

26.   Tosaki A, Maulik N, Cordis GA, Trifan OC, Popescu LM, Das DK. Ischemic preconditioning triggers phospholipase D signaling in the rat heart. Am J Physiol 1997; 273: H1860-H1866.

27.   Billah MM. Phospholipase D and cell signaling. Curr Opin Immunol 1993; 5: 114-123.

28.   Das DK, Engelman RM, Rousou JA, Breyer RH, Otani H, Lemeshow S. Role of membrane phospholipids in myocardial injury induced by ischemia and reperfusion. Am J Physiol 1986; 251: H71-H79.

29.   Moraru II, Jones RM, Popescu L, Engelman R, Das DK.Prazosin reduces myocardial ischemia/reperfusion-induced Ca2+ overloading in rat heart by inhibiting phosphoinositide signaling. Biochim Biophys Acta 1995; 1268: 1-8.

30.   Tosaki A, Maulik N, Engelman DT, Engelman RM, Das DK. The role of protein kinase C in ischemic/reperfused preconditioning isolated rat hearts. J Cardiovasc Pharmacol 1996; 28: 723-731.

31.   Fantl WJ, Johnson DE, Williams LT. Signalling by receptor tyrosine kinases. Ann Rev Biochem 1993; 62: 453-481.

32.   Meisenhelder J, Suh PG, Rhee SG, Hunter T. Phospholipase C gamma is substrate for the PDGF and EGF receptor protein tyrosine kinases in vivo and in vitro. Cell 1989; 57: 1109-1122.

33.   Ha KS, Exton JH. Differential translocation of protein kinase C isozymes by thrombin and platelet derived growth factor. A possible function for phosphatidylcholine-derived diacylglycerol. J Biol Chem 1993; 268: 10534-10539.

34.   Schmidt M, Huwe SM, Fasselt B et al. Mechanisms of phospholipase D stimulation by m3 muscarinic acetylcholine receptors. Evidence for involvement of tyrosine phosphorylation. Eur J. Biochem 1994; 225: 667-675.

35.   Rivard N, Rydzewska G, Lods JS, Martinex LJ, Morisset J. Pancreas growth , tyrosine kinase, PtdIns 3-kinase, and PLD involve gigh-affinity CCK-receptor occupation. Am J Physiol 1994; 266: G62-G70.

36.   Bourgoin S, Grinstein S. Peroxides of vanadate induce activation of phospholipase D in HL-60 cells. Role of tyrosine phosphorylation. J Biol Chem 1992; 267: 11908-11916.

37.   Fialkow L, Chan CK, Chan S, Grinstein S, Downey GP. Regulation of tyrosine phosphorylation in neutrophils by the NADPH oxidase. Role of reactive oxygen intermediates. J. Biol Chem 1993; 268: 17131-17137.

38.   Natarajan V, Scribner WM, Taher MM. 4-hydroxynonenal, a metabolite of lipid peroxidation, activates phospholipase D in vascular endothelial cells. Free Rad Biol Med 1993; 15: 365-375.

39.   Uings IJ, Thompson NT, Randall RW et al. Tyrosine phosphorylation is involved in receptor coupling to phospholipase D but not phospholipase C in the human neutrophil. Biochem J. 1992; 281: 597-600.

40.   Natarajan V, Vepa S, Verma RS, Scribner WM. Inhibitors of tyrosine kinases and protein tyrosine phosphatases modulate hydrogen peroxide-induced activation of endothelial cell phospholipase D. Am J Physiol (in press)

41.   Prasad MR, Jones RM. Enhanced membrane protein kinase C activity in myocardial ischemia. Basic Res Cardiol 1992; 87: 19-26.

42.   Henrich CJ, Simpson PC. Differential acute and chronic response of protein kinase C in cultured neonatal rat heart myocytes to a1-adrenergic and phorbol ester stimulation. J Mol Cell Cardiol 1988; 20: 1081-1085.

43.   Fearon CW, Tashjian AH. Thyrotropin-releasing hormone induces redistribution of protein kinase C in GH4C1 rat pitutary cells. J Biol Chem 1985; 260: 8366-8371.

44.   Ytrehus K, Liu Y, Downey JM. Preconditioning protects ischemic rabbit heart by protein kinase C activation Am J Physiol 1994; 266: H1145-H1152.

45.   Mitchell MB, Meng X, Brown J, Harken AH, Banerjee A. Preconditioning of isolated rat heart is mediated by protein kinase C activation. Am J. Physiol 1994; 266: H1145-H1152.

46.   Nishizuka Y. Studies and perspectives of protein kinase C. Science 1986; 233: 305-312.

47.   Maulik N, Sharma HS, Das DK. Induction of heme oxygenase gene expression during the reperfusion of ischemic rat myocardium. J Mol Cell Cardiol 1996; 28:1261-1270.

48.   Das DK, Engelman RM, Kimura Y. Molecular adaptation of cellular defences following preconditioning of the heart by repeated ischemia. Cardiovasc Res 1993; 27: 578-584.

49.   Brand T, Sharma HS, Fleischmann KE et al. Proto-oncogene expression in porcine myocardium subjected to ischemia and reperfusion. Circ Res 1992; 71: 1351-1360.

50.   Heads RJ, Latchman DS, Yellon DM. Differential stress protein mRNA expression during early ischemic preconditioning in the rabbit heart and its relationship to adenosine receptor function. J. Mol Cell Cardiol 1995; 27: 2133-2148.

51.   Bugge E, Ytrehus K. Ischemic preconditioning is protein kinase C dependent but not through stimulation of a adrenergic or adenosine receptors in the isolated rat heart. Cardiovas Res 1995; 29: 401-406.

52.   Dixon BS, Sharma RV, Dickerson T, Fortune J. Bradykinin and angiotensin II: activation of protein kinase C in arterial muscle. Am J Physiol. 1994; 266: C1406-C1420.

53.   Goto M, Liu Y, Yang XM, Ardell JL, Cohen MV, Downey JM. Role of bradykinin in protection of ischemic preconditioning in rabbit hearts. Circ Res 1995; 77: 611-621

54.   Liu Y, Tsuchida A, Cohen MV, Downey JM. Pretreatment with angiotensin II activates protein kinase C and limits myocardial infarction in isolated rabbit hearts. J Mol Cell Cardiol 1995; 27: 883-892.

55.   Yamazaki T, Komuro I, Kudoh S et al. Endothelin-1 is involved in mechanical stress-induced cardiomyocyte hypertrophy. J Biol Chem 1996; 271: 3221-3228.

56.   Lenormand P, Sardet C, Pages G, L'Allemain G, Brunet A, Pouyssegur J. Growth factors induce nuclear translocation of MAP kinases (p42 MAPK and p44 MAPK) but not of their activator MAP kinase kinase (p45 MAPK) in fibroblasts. J Cell Biol. 1993; 122,1079-1088.

57.   Force T, Bonventrem JV, Heidecker G, Rapp U, Avruch J, Kyriakis LM. Enzymatic characteristics of thew Raf-1 protein kinase. Proc Natl Acad Sci USA, 1994; 91: 1270-1274.

58.   Zu Y-L, Ai Y, Gilchrist A et al. High expression and activation of MAP kinase-activated protein kinase 2 in myocardium. J Mol Cell Cardiol 1997; 29: 2150-2168.

59.   Maulik N, Yoshida T, Zu Y-L, Das DK. Ischemic preconditioning triggers a tyrosine kinase-dependent signal transduction process involving 38P MAP kinases and MAPKAP kinase 2. J Mol Cell Cardiol 1997; 29: A272 (abstract).

60.   Egan SE, Weinberg, RA. The pathway to signal achievement. Nature 1993; 65: 781-783.

61.   Davis RJ. MPKs: new JNK expands the group. Trends Biochem Sci 1994; 19: 470-47.

62.   Raingeaud J, Whitmarsh AJ, Barrett T, Derijard B, Davies RJ. MKK3 and MKK6-regulated gene expression is mediated by the p38 mitogen-activated protein kinase signal transduction pathway. Mol Cell Biol 1996; 365: 781-783.

63.   Olson MF, Ashworth A, Hall A. An essential role for rho, rac and cdc 42 GTPases in cell cycle progression through GI. Science1995; 269: 1270-1272.

64.   Doza YN, Cuenda A, Thomas GM, Cohen P, Nebreda AR.Activation of the MAP kinase homologue RK requires the phosphorylation of Thr-180 & Thr-182 and both residues are phosphorylated in chemically stressed KB cells. FEBS Lett. 1995; 364: 223-228.

65.   Raingeaud J, Gupta S, Rogers J, Dickens M, Han J, Ulevitch RJ, Davis RJ. Pro-inflammatory cytokines and environmental stress cause p38 mitogen-activated

protein kinase activation by dual phosphorylation on tyrosine and threonine. J Biol Chem 1995; 270: 7420-7426.

66.   Raingeaud J, Whitmarsh AJ, Barrett T, Derijard B, Davis RJ. MKK3 & MKK6-regulated gene expression is mediated by the p38 mitogen-activated protein kinase signal transduction pathway. Mol Cell Biol 1996; 16: 1247-1255.

67.   Rouse J, Cohen P, Trigon S, Morange M, Alonso-Llamazares A, Zamanillo D, Hunt T, Nebreda AR. A novel kinase cascade triggered by stress and heat shock that stimulates MAPKAP kinase 2 and phosphorylation of the small heat shock proteins. Cell 1994; 78: 1027-1037.

68.   Lee JC, Laydon JT, McDonnell PC et al. A protein kinase involved in the regulation of inflammatory cytokine biosynthesis. Nature 1994; 372: 739-746.

69.   Derijard B, Raingeaud J, Barrett T et al. Independent human MAP-kinase signal transduction pathways defined by MEK and MKK isoforms. Science 1995; 267: 682-685.

70.   Han J, Lee JD, Bibbs L, Ulevitch RJ. A MAP kinase targeted by endotoxin and hyperosmolality in mammalian cells. Science 1994; 265: 808-811.

71.   Freshney NW, Rawlinson L, Guesdon F et al. Interleukin 1 activates a novel protein kinase cascade that results in the phosphorylation of HSP 27. Cell 1994; 78: 1039-1049.

72.   Ciocca DR, Oesterreich S, Chamness GC, McGuire WL, Fuqua SAW. Biological and clinical implications of heat shock protein 27000: a review. J Natl Cancer Inst 1993; 85: 1558-1570.

73.   Stokoe D, Engel K, Campbell DG, Cohen P, Gaeste M. Identification of MAPKAP kinase 2 as a major enzyme responsible for the phosphorylation of the small mammalian heat shock proteins. FEBS 1992; 313: 307-313.

74.   Zu YL, Ai Y, Gilchrist A, Labadia ME, Sha'afi RI, Huang CK. Activation of MAP kinase-activated protein kinase 2 in human neutrophils after phorbol ester or fMLP peptide stimulation. Blood 1996; 87: 5287-5296.

75.   Zu YL, Ai Y, Huang CK. Characterization of an autoinhibitory domain in human mitogen activated protein kinase activated protein kinase 2. J Biol Chem 1995; 270: 202-206.

76.   Maulik N, Wei ZJ, Engelman RM et al. Interleukin-1α preconditioning reduces myocardial ischemic reperfusion injury. Circulation 1993; 88: II387-394.

77.   Maulik N, Watanabe M, Engelman D et al. Myocardial adaptation to ischemia by oxidative stress induced by endotoxin. Am J Physiol 1995; 269: C907-C916.

78.   Landry J, Lambert H, Zhou M et al. Human HSP 27 is phosphorylated at serines 78 and 82 by heat shock and mitogen-activated kinases that recognize the same amino acid motif as S6 kinase II. J. Biol Chem 1992; 267: 794-803.

79.   Das DK, Maulik N, Engelman RM, Rousou JA, Deaton D, Flack JE. Signal transduction pathway leading to HSP 27 and HSP 70 gene expression during myocardial adaptation to stress. Ann N Y Acad Sci 1998; in press.

6

Changes in Cardiac Gene Expression After Ischaemia and Reperfusion

L V Mayne

1. Introduction

Physiological stress leads to the induction of new proteins that are important in mediating damage repair, affording protection from further insults or promoting cell injury and death. Identifying these proteins is an important first step towards understanding the molecular mechanisms underlying the stress response. As new or elevated protein synthesis can result from increased gene expression, studies of gene transcription provide a key to identifying proteins with important functions. In this chapter, the published data on genes that are transcriptionally up-regulated in cardiac tissue in response to ischaemia and reperfusion will be reviewed along with the transcription factors responsible for mediating the response and the known target genes. Ultimately, our interest is to understand the response of human myocardium to ischaemia and reperfusion, resulting from pathological conditions or surgery, and to understand the adaptive processes that may protect myocardial function. Few studies of gene transcription have, however, been conducted using human tissue, due to the limitations of working with living subjects. As a result, our understanding of the transcriptional response of myocardium to stress has been gained largely from animal and in vitro models. While these models have provided detailed biochemical and molecular data, the results must be interpreted with some caution.

2. Methodological Considerations

The validity of animal models of ischaemia-reperfusion for understanding the response of the human myocardium is suggested by comparative studies on their genomes. Sequencing and analysis of human and other mammalian genomes has demonstrated that gene structure and function are highly conserved between different species, consistent with the conservation of biochemical pathways and cellular responses between species. However, significant species differences do exist in the structure and expression of genes and the biochemical pathways in which they operate. Thus, data from animal studies must be considered only as a paradigm for the response of the human heart. In addition to the variety of species, numerous different protocols for ischaemia-reperfusion are employed, ranging from in vivo treatment of anaesthetised whole animals, manipulation of excised intact hearts to isolated cells in culture. These models vary greatly in their complexity and ability to reproduce naturally occurring events. Whole animal studies most closely model the complexity of the in vivo situation, while cells in culture offer the simplest system and controlled conditions. In each case, the data must be interpreted within the limitations of the system used.

The molecular basis of the cellular response to other forms of stress, such as ionising and ultra-violet (UV) radiation [1] and hyperthermia [2], has been studied in great detail and several key concepts regarding the stress response, relevant to this review, have emerged. In particular, many aspects of the stress-response pathway appear to be conserved between different stressors. One reason for this may be that different external stimuli produce overlapping forms of intracellular damage; for example, radiation, hyperthermia and anoxia-reoxygenation all generate reactive oxygen species. Another consideration is that programmed cell death occurs by a highly conserved pathway, and one aspect of protection against injury may be blocking or delaying cell death to permit cellular repair. As the cell death pathway is conserved, the mechanisms by which protection may be afforded may also be conserved and limited.

3. Pathophysiological Considerations

By its very nature, ischaemia and reperfusion of tissue generates a complex pattern of stresses and cell responses. The heart is composed of muscle, connective and vascular tissue and is perfused by a range of blood cells, including lymphocytes, macrophages, and neutrophils. Although many aspects of the stress response, such as detection of damage and the intracellular signalling cascades, are very similar between different cell types, the final response of each cell type will reflect, to some degree, their specialised function. During ischaemia, restriction of the blood supply creates an oxygen deficit leading to anaerobic respiration, with depletion of ATP pools and a build up of waste products, such as carbon dioxide [3]. Metabolic processes, dependent on ATP for energy become vulnerable, and both the contractile function of the myocyte, which requires ATP for the calcium-fluxes that regulate contraction, and mitochondrial respiration, are particularly sensitive. Restoration of the blood supply restores oxygen to the tissue, but regeneration of ATP stores is slow. Reperfusion also brings the return of immune system cells, with a concomitant inflammatory response and free radical production that leads to oxidant stress. Additional free radicals are generated through disruption of mitochondrial respiration.

4. Examination of Gene Regulation

The published data reporting the induction or up-regulation of genes, following ischaemia and reperfusion in a variety of cardiac models, is presented in Table 1, but members of the heat shock protein (HSP) gene family have been excluded, as these are discussed in greater detail in chapter 7. A brief description of the model system used in the published work, the ischaemia-reperfusion protocol followed and the method used to assess gene expression are also included. The majority of published studies examining gene expression following ischaemia-reperfusion used excised rat hearts or live anaesthetised pigs. However, no consistent experimental approach was followed and a wide variety of ischaemia-reperfusion protocols were used. This review will not focus on the experimental variability between these studies, but will consider the data in a wider context to establish the potential role of these genes in the response to ischaemia-reperfusion.

The most commonly used methods for establishing expression levels of genes are summarised in Table 2. These methods [5, 6] either examine the mRNA transcript of the gene or the protein product, and each method provides qualitatively different information. There are several mechanisms whereby protein activity and function can be increased, including increased transcription of the gene. The availability of rapid and relatively simple molecular techniques for studying RNA has focused attention on RNA transcription as a rapid screen for identifying changes in protein expression. In the majority of cases, increased transcription rates lead to the accumulation of mRNAs and more protein is produced as a consequence. However, this is not always the case, and it therefore remains necessary to confirm that observed changes in transcription rates or the increased levels of mRNA do lead to changes in protein activity.

The genes presented in Table 1 were, in almost all cases, initially identified in another context, and their expression was then examined in a model of ischaemia-reperfusion. These genes do not, therefore, represent a random sampling of genes reflecting the variety of underlying molecular processes; they are the result of targeted analysis of known genes. More recent studies [7, 80] have begun to use molecular approaches such as subtractive hybridisation and differential display, which offer an unbiased approach to the study of altered gene expression and will provide a more representative picture of the molecular pathways implicated in the stress response.

For clarity of discussion, the genes listed in Table 1 are broadly divided into five categories: transcription factors; cytokines and growth factors; sarcoplasmic reticulum calcium release channel and calcium-handling proteins; antioxidants; and miscellaneous. The discussion will evaluate the data presented in Table 1 in the context of other published work, with the following points in mind:

1. is there evidence that the protein is consistently up-regulated in response to ischaemia-reperfusion?
2. is the known function of the protein compatible with a role in the response to stress?
3. is the protein involved in other stress-responses?

5. Transcription Factors

The transcription factors, c-fos, erg-1, ATF3 and c-myc and members of the jun family are reported to be transcriptionally up-regulated following ischaemia-reperfusion in a variety of models [8-15]. Expression is both rapid and transient and forms the so-called 'immediate-early response' to stress. These transcription factors recognise and bind to specific DNA sequences found in the regulatory regions of target genes and promote their transcription. The number of potential target genes for these transcription factors is large, and the pattern of genes induced will be determined by a host of other factors, including the expression and activity of other transcription factors. In this way, the same stress-induced transcription factors can give rise to cell type and stress-specific responses.

c-Fos, Jun and ATF3

On its own, c-fos is unable to bind DNA and its transciptional activity is dependent on its interaction with members of the jun family [16]. Together, with ATF, these proteins form the AP1 transcription factor, which may be composed of either jun:jun homodimers, fos:jun heterodimers or ATF:jun heterodimers [17]. Levels of AP1 are normally low in unstimulated cells, as are the levels of jun family members, but AP1 activity is consistently induced following stimulation with a wide range of growth factors and physiological stresses. The activity of the AP1 complex is further regulated by changes in phosphorylation, through both the protein kinase C pathway and the stress activated protein kinases (SAPK) [15].

c-Myc

c-myc is a member of the basic helix-loop-helix leucine-zipper (bHLHZ) transcription factor family and plays an important role in cell proliferation, transformation, differentiation and apoptosis [18]. The transcriptional activity of c-myc is dependent on its dimerisation with MAX, another bHLHZ protein and the heterodimers bind with high affinity to the E-box-related sequnces to promote transcription. MAX is also able to form homodimers or heterodimers with other proteins such as MAD and MIZ-1 [19, 20].

Though at least three reports demonstrated induction of c-myc mRNA following ischaemia-reperfusion [9, 12, 21], three other reports failed to show induction using similar methodologies [10, 11, 13]. The induction of c-myc mRNA in rat proximal tubular epithelial cells following oxidative stress in vitro [22] is consistent with a role in the response to oxidative stress. However, the data supporting c-myc induction following stress is controversial and is further complicated by the observation that, for at least one form of stress (heat shock), the half-life of c-myc mRNA was increased, leading to greater stability and consequently elevated levels of the RNA [23, 24] independent of any effect on transcription. Therefore, in the absence of studies which unequivocally demonstrate induction of the protein, the role of c-myc in mediating the response to ischaemia-reperfusion remains unclear.

Egr-1

Both Plumier et al [8] and Brand et al [11] demonstrated induction of the early growth response-1 (egr-1) gene following ischaemia-reperfusion. Few studies have examined the role of egr-1 in a context specifically relevant to ischaemia-reperfusion in the heart, and our knowledge of egr-1 function comes from studies in other contexts. A role in apoptosis was demonstrated for egr-1 by stimuli that elevate intracellular calcium and the effect of egr-1 appeared to be mediated through a p53 dependent pathway [25]. Egr-1 was also implicated in the synthesis and secretion of transforming growth factor β (TGF-β) [26]. The TGF-β gene promoter contains egr-1 DNA binding sites, consistent with the idea that egr-1 regulates TGF-β gene expression [26]. TGF-β, itself, was reported to be expressed in response to ischaemia-reperfusion (see Table 1 for references). The significance of TGF-β expression in ischaemia-reperfusion will be discussed below. Transcription of egr-1 may be sensitive to the redox state of the cell and may be regulated as part of the inflammatory response to tissue damage, as its expression was induced

Table1: Genes up-regulated in models of cardiac ischaemia-reperfusion

GENE	REFERENCE	SPECIES	TREATMENT[1,2]	METHOD
TRANSCRIPTION FACTORS				
c-fos	Plumier et al 1996[8]	Rat - excised heart	30' i x 30', 60', or 90' r	In situ hybridisation
	Wechsler et al 1994[9,10]	Rat - excised heart	5-20' i + 0-120' r	Slot blot ant northern analysis
	Brand et al 1992[11]	Pig - anaesthetised	(10' i x 30' r) x 2	Northern analysis
	Das et al 1993[12], 1994[80]	Rat - excised heart	5' i x 70' r	Northern analysis
	Sharma et al 1992[13]	Pig - anaesthetised	(10' i x 30 ' r) x 2	RT-PCR, Northern analysis
	Peng et al 1995[14]	Rat neonatal cardiomyocytes in vitro	hydrogen peroxide	Northern analysis, Immunohistochemistry
c-jun	Plumier et al 1996[8]	Rat - excised heart	30' i x 30', 60', or 90' r	In situ hybridisation
	Knoll et al 1994[21]	Pig - anaesthetised	(10' i x 30' r) (10' i) x 30', 60' or 90' r	Nuclear run-on with cardiomyocytes
	Brand et al 1992[11]	Pig - anaesthetised	(10' i x 30' r) x 2	Northern analysis
	Peng et al 1995[14]	Rat neonatal cardiomyocytes in vitro	hydrogen peroxide	Northern analysis, Immunohistochemistry
	Yin et al 1997[15]	Rat - excised heart	(20' or 45' i)+ 30' r	In situ hybridisation
jun-B	Knoll et al 1994[21]	Pig - anaesthetised	(10' i x 30' r) (10' i) x 30', 60' or 90' r	Nuclear run-on with cardiomyocytes
	Brand et al 1992[11]	Pig - anaesthetised	(10' i x 30' r) x 2	Northern analysis
jun-D	Knoll et al 1994[21]	Pig - anaesthetised	(10' i x 30' r) (10' i) x 30', 60' or 90' r	Nuclear run-on with cardiomyocytes
ATF3	Yin et al 1997[15]	Rat - excised heart	(20' or 45' i)+ 30' r	In situ hybridisation
egr - 1	Plumier et al 1996[8]	Rat - excised heart	30' i x 30', 60', 90' r	In situ hybridisation
	Brand et al 1992[11]	Pig - anaesthetised	(10' i x 30' r) x 2	Northern analysis
c-myc	Knoll et al 1994[21]	Pig - anaesthetised	(10' i x 30' r) (10' i) x 30', 60' or 90' r	Nuclear run-on with cardiomyocytes
	Das et al 1993[12]	Rat - excised heart	5' i x 70' r	Northern analysis
	Weschler et al 1994[10]	Rat - excised heart	5-20' i + 0-120' r	Slot blot

Table 1. continued

CYTOKINES and GROWTH FACTORS				
IL-6	Chandrasekar et al 1997[32]	Rat - open chest	15' i x 1h or 3h r	Northern and Western blotting
	Yamauchi - Takihara et al 1995[47]	Rat neonatal cardiomyocytes in vitro	hypoxia / reoxygenation	Northern analysis
IL-2	Herskowitz et al 1995[33]	Rat - anaesthetised	35' i + various r times	RT-PCR and Western blotting
Il-1ß	Chandrasekar et al 1997[32]	Rat - open chest	15' i x 1h or 3h r	Northern and Western blotting
	Herskowitz et al 1995[33]	Rat - anaesthetised	35' i + various r times	RT-PCR and Western blotting
TNF-α	Chandrasekar et al 1997[32]	Rat - open chest	15' i x 1h or 3h r	Northern and Western blotting
	Herskowitz et al 1995[33]	Rat - anaesthetised	35' i + various r times	RT-PCR and Western blotting
	Gurevitch et al 1996[34]	Rat - excised heart	cardioplegic arrest, 1 h global ischaemia, 30' reperfusion	ELISA on reperfusion effluent
TGF-β1	Herskowitz et al 1995[33]	Rat - anaesthetised	35' i + various r times	RT-PCR and Western blotting
	Sharma et al 1992[13]	Pig - anaesthetised	chronic coronary artery occlusion	RT-PCR, Northern analysis In situ hybridisation
TGF-ß 1,2,3	Flanders et al 1993[57]	Neonatal rat cardiomyocytes in vitro + in vivo	hyperthermia	Northern analysis and immunoprecipitation/gel analysis of protein
IGF-II	Kluge et al 1995[61]	Pig - anaesthetised	(10' i x 30' r) x 2	In situ hybridisation
IGFBP-5	Kluge et al 1995[61]	Pig - anaesthetised	(10' i x 30' r) x 2	In situ hybridisation
HBGF-1 (aFGF)	Sharma et al 1992[13]	Pig - anaesthetised	Chronic coronary artery occlusion	RT-PCR, Northern analysis In situ hybridisation

Table 1. continued

CALCIUM REGULATING PROTEINS			
Ca^{+2} ATPase	Frass et al 1993[74]	Pig - anaethetised	10' i + r + 10' i +90'r	Northern analysis
	Knoll et al 1994[21]	Pig - anaesthetised	(10' i x 30' r) (10' i) x 30', 60' or 90' r	Nuclear run-on with cardiomyocytes
Calmodulin	Knoll et al 1994[21]	Pig - anaesthetised	(10' i x 30' r) (10' i) x 30', 60' or 90' r	Nuclear run-on with cardiomyocytes
Phospholamban	Knoll et al 1994[21]	Pig - anaesthetised	(10' i x 30' r) (10' i) x 30', 60' or 90' r	Nuclear run-on with cardiomyocytes
	Frass et al 1993[74]	Pig - anaethetised	10' i + r + 10' i +90'r	Northern analysis
Calsequestrin	Knoll et al 1994[21]	Pig - anaesthetised	(10' i x 30' r) (10' i) x 30', 60' or 90' r	Nuclear run-on with cardiomyocytes
	Frass et al 1993[74]	Pig - anaethetised	10' i + r + 10' i +90'r	Northern analysis
ANTIOXIDANTS			
Mn-SOD	Chandrasekar et al 1997[32]	Rat - open chest	15' i x 1h or 3hr	Northern and Western blotting
	Das et al 1993[12], 1994[80]	Rat - excised heart	5' i x 70' r	Northern analysis
Catalase	Das et al 1993[12], 1994[80]	Rat - excised heart	5' i x 70' r	Northern analysis
	Chandrasekar et al 1997[32]	Rat - open chest	15' i x 1h or 3hr	Northern and Western blotting
Glutathione peroxidase	Chandrasekar et al 1997[32]	Rat - open chest	15' i x 1h or 3hr	Northern and Western blotting
Heme oxygenase	Sharma et al 1996[42]	Pig - anaesthetised	(10' i x 30' r) + 10' i x 30,90' or 210'	Dot blot and Northern Analysis

Table 1. continued

MISCELLANEOUS

Cytochrome oxidases I,II,III	Das et al 1994[80]	Rat - excised heart	1x or 4 x (5'i x 10'r) + 60'r	Cloned by cDNA subtraction
ATPase 6 and 8	Das et al 1994[80]	Rat - excised heart	1x or 4 x (5'i x 10'r) + 60'r	Cloned by cDNA subtraction
Cytochrome b	Das et al 1994[80]	Rat - excised heart	1x or 4 x (5'i x 10'r) + 60'r	Cloned by cDNA subtraction
FAT	Maulik + Das 1996[7]	Rat - excised heart	i, (5' i x 10'r) x 4	Northern analysis
		Rat - excised heart	5-20' i + 0-120' r	Northern analysis
Ubiquitin	Knoll et al 1994[21]	Pig - anaesthetised	(10' i x 30' r) (10' i) x 30', 60' or 90' r	Nuclear run-on with cardiomyocytes
	Andres et al 1993[79]	Pig - anaesthetised	(10' i x 30' r) x 2	Slot blot, Northern analysis, Nuclear run-on, Western blotting
	Sharma et al 1996[42]	Pig - anaesthetised	(10' i x 30' r) + 10' i x 30,90' or 210'	Dot blot and Northern analysis
PAI - 1	Knoll et al 1994[21]	Pig - anaesthetised	(10' i x 30' r) (10' i) x 30', 60' or 90' r	Nuclear run-on with cardiomyocytes
GAPDH	Knoll et al 1994[21]	Pig - anaesthetised	(10' i x 30' r) (10' i) x 30', 60' or 90' r	Nuclear run-on with cardiomyocytes
Tissue factor	Golino et al 1996[35]	Rabbit - anaesthetised	5'i x 2 h r	In vitro activity of protein

1. i = period of ischaemia; r = period of reperfusion
2. In vitro experiments using cultured cardiomyocytes treated with hypoxia, anoxia and hydrogen peroxide are included as supporting data.

by hydrogen peroxide and by proinflammatory cytokines. These data together support the role of egr-1 in mediating the response to ischaemia-reperfusion.

HSF-1 and NFκB

Two other transcription factors play an important role in the response to ischaemia/reperfusion; heat shock factor 1 (HSF-1), which is the primary transcription factor involved in the induction of the heat shock family of proteins and NF kappa B (NFkB). However, in contrast to the transcription factors discussed above, both HSF-1 and NFkB are constitutively expressed, but in an inactive form, and their ability to promote transcription is induced following many types of stress.

In unstressed cells, HSF-1 is primarily a monomer located in both the cytoplasm and nucleus and is functionally inactive [27] Following physiological stress, such as ischaemia-reperfusion, HSF-1 trimerises and is phosphorylated. These trimers are translocated to the nucleus, where they bind to the heat shock element of HSP promoters activating transcription. Early studies suggested that HSF-1 activity might be negatively regulated [28] and HSP70 has been implictated in this role as in vitro studies demonstrated its binding to the active form of HSF-1 and exogenous HSP70 prevents activation of HSF-1 in vivo [29].

NFkB is found in the cytoplasm of unstimulated cells in a complex with the inhibitory protein, IkB [30]. Activation of NFkB occurs when phosphorylation of IkB leads to dissociation of the NFkB:IkB complex and degradation of IkB. NFkB is then released and translocated to the nucleus. Activation of NFkB is triggered by proinflammatory cytokines, phorbol esters, lipopolysaccharide, UV and ionising-radiation and other stressors, which generate reactive oxygen species (ROS) [14]. ROS are believed to be the intracellular messenger that leads to NFkB activation, probably through the action of a redox sensitive protein kinase.

6. Cytokines and Growth Factors

Tumour necrosis factor alpha (TNF-α), interleukin 1 beta (IL-1β) and interleukin 6 (IL-6) are proinflammatory cytokines expressed rapidly in response to environmental stress and are proposed to play a role in mediating the myocardial response to tissue injury [31]. TNF-α and IL-1β also have well-defined roles in programmed cell death.

TNF-α

Increased gene transcription and synthesis and secretion of TNF-α protein, following cardiac ischaemia-reperfusion, has been demonstrated in a number of model systems [32-34] and in plasma from patients suffering from acute myocardial infarction, complicated by heart failure [36]. The ability of anti-TNF-α antibodies to improve myocardial recovery following ischaemia-reperfusion in the isolated rat heart suggested a deleterious role for TNF-α in myocardial function [37]. However, studies of brain ischaemia in transgenic mice lacking the TNF-α receptors demonstrated an increased sensitivity to brain ischaemia, suggesting that TNF-α may have beneficial effects at least in neurones (reviewed in reference 38).

TNF-α induces oxidant stress through the generation of ROS from the mitochondrial respiratory chain and this contributes to its cytotoxic effects. It is also able to affect gene expression through a number of pathways including AP1-dependent transcription [39], NFkB activation and MAPK [40], leading to induction of jun [41]. c-fos, HSP27 [42], HSP72 [43], HSP70, glutathione [39], manganese dependent superoxide dismutase (Mn-SOD) [44, 45], ubiquitin [13] and synthesis of IL-1 and IL-6 [40] in target cells. Another important role of TNF-α is to facilitate neutrophil migration across the vascular wall and to stimulate activation of neutrophils. Activated neutrophils generate ROS and may be the principal effector cells of reperfusion injury [46]. TNF-α may, therefore, be an important mediator of reperfusion injury.

IL-6

Few studies have examined the induction of IL-6 in the heart following ischaemia-reperfusion [32], but other studies provided data consistent with a role for IL-6 in the response to stress. IL-6 mRNA and/or protein levels were reported to increase following hypoxia-reoxygenation of isolated cardiomyocytes [47] following localised or whole body hyperthermia in the rat and following X-irradiation of HeLa cells [49]. IL-6 was also reported to promote transcription of HSP90 via MAPK and SAPK-dependent pathways [50]. Exogenous IL-6, when added to HeLa cultures, induced expression of Mn-SOD.

IL-1β

IL-1β has only recently been identified as a stress-response gene in the heart [32,33]. Previous studies demonstrated induction of IL1-β mRNA following anoxia of neurones cultured in vitro [51] and following hyperthermia in the rat in vivo [48]. IL-1β also induced activation of the MAPK and SAPK [52] and expression of metallothionein IIA [53] and glutathione peroxidase [54].

TGF-β

TGF-β1, TGF-β2 and TGF-β3 belong to a family of closely related cytokines, with pleiotropic functions that are often dependent on their local concentration and context (reviewed in reference 55). TGF-β can regulate proliferation, expression of extra-cellular matrix proteins, promote angiogenesis and wound healing. It has both pro- and anti-inflammatory activities and can antagonise lymphocyte and macrophage functions. TGF-β regulates gene transcription through the MAD family of transcription factors and genes which are reported to be targets of TGF-β include: c-myc, collagen, fibronectin, c-jun, junB, c-fos and various growth factors. Functional studies also demonstrated the ability of TGF-β to regulate the beat rate of rat neonatal myocytes in culture [55].

The data presented in Table 1 are consistent with the induction of TGF-β following prolonged or chronic ischaemia, and TGF-β is likely to be a general stress-response protein as its induction was also reported in human fibroblasts following hypoxia [57] and after hyperthermia in both isolated rat cardiomyocytes and whole heart [58]. Exogenous TGF-β was able to provide protection against ischaemia-reperfusion injury in several species [59-61] supporting a role for TGF-β in ischaemia-reperfusion, possibly in the adaptation to stress. In view of the induction of pro-inflammatory cytokines following ischaemia-reperfusion (see Table 1), and the involvement of TNF-α and IL-1β in programmed cell death, the role of TGF-β may be in modulating the inflammatory response, protecting the tissue from the potentially deleterious effects of these cytokines. TGF-β may also play a role in promoting wound healing following ischaemia-reperfusion.

IGF-II

Only one study has reported the expression of insulin-like growth factor II (IGF-II) following ischaemia in the heart [62]. This report also demonstrated the induction of the insulin growth factor binding protein 5 (IGFBP5). IGF-I and IGFBP5 were shown previously to be co-ordinately regulated following hypoxia-ischaemia in the brain [63]. The ischaemia-reperfusion protocol that was used by Kluge et al [62] induced preconditioning or adaptation to ischaemia, suggesting that IGF-II/IGFBP5 may be involved in this process. Consistent with this finding are two subsequent reports [64, 65], including one from an independent group, that demonstrated the ability of exogenously administered IGF-II to protect against myocardial infarction after ischaemia. The data on IGF-II are too limited to draw firm conclusions, but IGF-II is a good candidate for a protein involved in adaptation to ischaemia.

Table 2:   Common Methods for the Study of Gene Expression

METHOD[1]	END POINT
Slot blot	Number of RNA transcripts
Northern analysis	Number of RNA transcripts Size of transcript Identifies splice variants
RNA protection assays	Number of RNA transcripts
In situ hybridisation	Identifies site of mRNA expression and provides crude measurement of RNA levels
RT-PCR or competitive PCR	Rapid method for quantifying the number of RNA transcripts, can detect alternative splice variants only when splice-specific primers are used.
Nuclear run-on	In vitro synthesis of RNA from isolated nuclei, indicates genes being actively transcribed and relative levels of RNA synthesis
Western blotting	Quantifies amount of protein Size of protein Alternative or processed forms
ELISA	Semi-quantitative measurement of protein Useful for very small quantities
Immunohistochemistry	Antibody-based technique for visualisation of protein expression in cells or tissues. Not quantitative

1. For details on these methods see Sambrook et al. [5] and Harlow and Lane [6].

HBGF-1 (aFGF)

Heparin binding growth factor-1 is more commonly known as acidic fibroblast growth factor (aFGF). The role of aFGF in the response to ischaemia/reperfusion has been poorly studied and conclusions cannot be drawn. However, it is of interest to note that aFGF administered to rats was reported to protect against ischaemia-reperfusion injury in the heart [66].

7. Sarcoplasmic Reticulum Calcium Regulating Proteins

Calcium release from the sarcoplasmic reticulum (SR) is critical for the initiation of cardiac muscle contraction and the SR also plays a role in sequestering calcium to allow muscle relaxation (reviewed in reference 67). Calcium is stored within the SR through the action of a calcium and ATP-dependent pump, which is regulated by the phosphorylation of the SR membrane protein, phospholamban. Calcium release into the cytosol is regulated by the SR calcium release channel (ryanodine receptor). The calcium-binding protein, calsequestrin, operates within the SR lumen and may function to regulate the calcium channel [68].

The activity of both the calcium and ATP-dependent pump and the SR calcium release channel is sensitive to ROS. The channel is activated by free radicals in a calmodulin-dependent mechanism, resulting in an efflux of calcium from the SR into the cytosol [69-71]. Both pre-ischaemic calcium-loading of isolated rat hearts and low calcium haemodialysis in the dog were shown to protect against myocardial ischaemia-reperfusion injury [72, 73]. These data are consistent with the SR calcium release channel and calcium and ATP-dependent pump being a target for ischaemia-reperfusion injury.

The data from Table 1 [21, 74] suggest that ischaemia-reperfusion leads to up-regulation of mRNA for the SR calcium dependent ATPase and several calcium-binding proteins. However, few data are available to correlate mRNA levels with improved function. In patients with end stage heart failure due to ischaemic cardiomyopathy and idiopathic dilated cardiomyopathy, there is a reduction in mRNA levels for phospholamban and the calcium-dependent ATPase, however, the reduction in mRNA levels was not accompanied by changes in protein levels [75, 76] Therefore, while calcium fluxes are implicated in ischaemia-reperfusion injury and the function of the SR calcium release channel and pump are sensitive to oxidative damage, further work is required to establish whether the changes in transcription effect changes in calcium handling.

8. Antioxidants

The induction of proteins with the ability to scavenge free radicals is a well-characterised response to oxidative stress. The data in Table 1 and the wide literature on antioxidant changes following stress are consistent with their role in protecting against free radical damage produced during ischaemia-reperfusion. A full discussion is beyond the scope of this chapter but for a detailed discussion see reference 77, and also refer to chapter 8.

9. Miscellaneous

Ubiquitin

Ubiquitin is a well-described stress-induced protein with a role in protein degradation [78]. The data reported in Table 1 [21, 79] are consistent with the upregulation of ubiquitin following ischaemia-reperfusion. Data on the remaining genes in Table 1 are limited, and defining the role of these genes in ischaemia-reperfusion requires considerable further work. Only a few brief points on selected genes will be mentioned.

Enzymes of the Mitochondrial Respiratory Chain

A single report [80] examines mitochondrial mRNA after ischaemia in the heart. Prolonged depletion of ATP leads to mitochondrial dysfunction, calcium overload and free radical production, and components of the respiratory chain are lost or denatured [4]. Restoration of these components by new synthesis may be part of the recovery process.

Fatty Acid Transport (Fat) Gene

The protein encoded by the Fat gene (also known as CD36) was implicated in membrane binding and transport of long-chain fatty acids, which are a major energy substrate in the heart [81]. Reduced long-chain fatty acid uptake and a deficiency in CD36 was demonstrated in patients with some types of hypertrophic cardiomyopathy [82].

Plasminogen Activator Inhibitor-1 (PAI-1)

Proteolysis is an important part of the inflammatory process and stress leads to the induction of proteases (e.g. see Miskin and Reich [83]). Induction of PAI-1 may play a role in suppressing inflammation following ischaemia-reperfusion. PAI is also induced by TGF-β, which is itself regulated by egr-1, all of which are reported to be upregulated following ischaemia-reperfusion (see Table 1).

10. Perspective and Conclusion

This review has examined the reported changes in gene transcription and protein synthesis, seen in a wide variety of ischaemia-reperfusion models. For convenience, the heat shock family of proteins were considered separately in another chapter and this review is necessarily biased to those genes not traditionally considered as heat shock proteins. A further bias exists in the way that researchers have selected genes for analysis of their role in ischaemia-reperfusion. In almost every case, the genes examined were chosen because they were previously identified as stress-response genes, in other contexts, or because their proteins function in pathways known to be sensitive to ischaemia and reperfusion injury. Despite these short-comings, a number of important conclusions and predictions can be made from the data presented here.

An immediate response to ischaemia-reperfusion is the induction or activation of a range of transcription factors including AP1, egr-1, HSF-1 and NFkB. The diversity of these factors and the large number of potential target genes regulated by their activities, suggests many more genes are involved in the cellular response to ischaemia-reperfusion and remain to be identified.

The identification of numerous cytokines and growth factors as stress-response genes in the heart emphasises the important role of the inflammatory response in mediating both injury and repair induced by ischaemia and reperfusion. However, while the mechanisms leading to cell death and further tissue injury by cytokines are at least partly understood, evidence suggests they also have a poorly understood role in protecting damaged tissue. The ability of the anti-inflammatory cytokine TGF-β to both suppress or modulate the immune response, as well as to protect against damage, suggests that the balance between pro- and anti-inflammatory cytokines may be an important determinant of eventual tissue damage or recovery.

The function of both the SR and mitochondria are essential to the specialised function of the cardiomyocyte, and both are highly sensitive to damage by ROS, an important stressor generated by ischaemia-reperfusion. The limited data presented here suggests that changes in the expression of genes, whose function is associated with these organelles, may play a role in ischaemia-reperfusion and are potential candidates for further study.

The data presented in this chapter suggest that the response to ischaemia-reperfusion is diverse and involves numerous different metabolic processes, many of which may not yet have been identified in this connection. The recent development of improved molecular techniques [84, 85] for the rapid and anonymous identification of changes in gene expression will open the way towards a fuller understanding of the underlying cellular processes that represent the response to ischaemia-reperfusion.

Acknowledgements

Work in the author's laboratory is supported by the Brighton Heart Support Trust, the R M Phillips Charitable Foundation and the Medical Research Council. The author would like to thank Dr R Killick for helpful comments and suggestions on the manuscript.

References

1.   Trautinger F, Kindas-Mugge, Knobler RM, Honigsmann HJ. Stress proteins in the cellular response to ultraviolet radiation. Photochem Photobiol B 1996; 35: 141-148.

2.   Morimoto RI, Sarge KD, Abravaya K. Transcriptional regulation of heat shock genes - a paradigm for inducible genomic responses. J Biol Chem 1992; 267: 21987-21990.

3.   Maxwell SR, Lip GY. Reperfusion injury: a review of the pathophysiology, clinical manifestations and therapeutic options. Int J Cardiol 1997; 58: 95-117.

4.   Piper HM, Noll T, Siegmund B. Mitochondrial function in the oxygen depeleted and reoxygenated myocardial cell. Cardiovasc Res 1994; 28: 1-15.

5.   Sambrook J, Fritsch EF, Maniatis T. Molecular Cloning: A laboratory manual, second edition, 1989. Cold Spring Harbor Laboratory Press.

6.   Harlow E, Lane D. Antibodies: A laboratory manual, 1988 Cold Spring Harbor Laboratory Press.

7.   Maulik N, Das DK. Molecular cloning, sequencing and expression analysis of a fatty acid transport gene in rat heart induced by ischemic preconditioning and oxidative stress. Mol Cell Biochem 1996; 160/161: 241-247.

8.   Plumier J-C L, Robertson H A, Currie RW. Differential accumulation of mRNA for immediate early genes and heat shock genes in heart after ischaemic injury. J Mol Cell Cardiol 1996; 28: 1251-1260.

9.   Wechsler AS, Entwistle JC, Yeh T, Ding M, Jakoi ER. Early gene changes in mycardial ischemia. Ann Thorac Surg 1994; 58: 1282-1284.

10.   Wechsler AS, Entwistle JWC, Ding M, Yeh T, Jakoi ER. Myocardial stunning: association with altered gene expression. J Card Surg 1994; 9: 537-542.

11.   Brand T, Sharma HS, Fleischmann KE et al. Proto-oncogene expression in porcine myocardium subjected to ischaemia and reperfusion. Circ Res 1992; 71: 1351-1360.

12.   Das DK, Engleman RM, Kimura Y. Molecular adaption of cellular defences following preconditioning of the heart by repeated ischemia. Cardiovasc Res 1993; 27: 578-584.

13.   Sharma HS, Wunsch M, Brand T, Verdouw PD, Schaper W. Molecular-biology of the coronary vascular and myocardial responses to ischemia. J Cardiovasc Pharmacol 1992; 20: S23-S31.

14.   Peng M, Huang L, Xie ZJ, Huang WH, Askari A. Oxidant-induced activations of nuclear factor-kappa B and activator protein-1 in cardiac myocytes. Cell Mol Biol Res 1995; 41: 189-97.

15.   Yin T, Sandhur G, Wolfgang CD et al. Tissue specific pattern of stress kinase activation in ischaemia reperfused heart and kidney. J Biol Chem 1997; 272: 19943-19950.

16.   Chiu R, Boyle WJ, Meek J, Smeal T, Hunter T, Karin M. The c-fos protein interacts with c-Jun/AP1 to stimulate transcription of AP1 responsive genes. Cell 1988; 54: 541-552.

17.   Karin M, Liu Zg, Zandi E. AP-1 function and regulation. Curr Opin Cell Biol 1997; 9: 240-246.

18.   Marcu KB, Bossone SA, Patel AJ. Myc function and regulation. Ann Rev Biochem 1992; 61: 809-860.

19.   Peukert K, Staller P, Schneider A, Carmichael G, Hanel F, Eilers M. An alternative pathway for gene regulation by Myc. EMBO J 1997; 16: 5672-5686.

20.   Ayer DE, Eisenman RN. A switch from Myc:Max to Mad:Max heterocomplexes accompanies monocyte/macrophage differentiation. Genes Dev 1993; 7: 2110-2119.

21.   Knoll R, Arras M, Zimmermann R, Schaper J, Schaper W. Changes in gene expression following short coronary occlusions studied in porcine hearts with run-on assays. Cardiovasc Res 1994; 28: 1062-1069.

22.   Maki A, Berezesku IK, Fargnli J, Holbrook NJ, Trump BF. Role of $[Ca^{2+}]i$ in induction of c-fos, c-jun and c-myc RNA in rat PTE after oxidative stress. FASEB J 1992; 6: 919-924.

23.   Bukh AM, Martinez-Valdez H, Freedman SJ, Freedman MH, Cohen A. The expression of c-fos, c-jun and c-myc genes is regulated by heat shock in human lymphoid cells. J Immunol 1990; 144: 4835-4840.

24.   Sadis S, Hickey E, Weber LA. Effect of heat shock on RNA metabolism in HeLa cells. J Cell Physiol 1988; 135: 377-386.

25.   Nair P, Muthukkumar S, Sells SF, Han SS, Sukhatme VP, Rangnekar VM. Early growth response-1-dependent apoptosis is mediated by p53. J Biol Chem 1997; 272: 20131-20138.

26.   Liu C, Calogero A, Adamson E, Mercola D. Egr-1, the reluctant suppression factor: Egr-1 is known to function in the regulation of growth, differentiation, and also has significant tumor suppressor activity and a mechanism involving the induction of TGF-beta 1 is postulated to account for this suppressor activity. Crit Rev Oncog 1996; 7: 101-125.

27.   Baler R, Dahl G, Voellmy R. Activation of heat shock gene transcription by heat shock factor 1 is accompanied by oligomerisation, modification, and rapid translocation of heat shock transcription factor HSF1. Mol Cell Biol 1993; 13: 2486-2496.

28.   Sarge KD, Murphy SP, Morimoto RI. Activation of heat shock gene transcription by heat shock factor 1 involves oligomerisation, acquisition of DNA-binding activity, and nuclear localisation and can occur in the absence of stress. Mol Cell Biol 1993; 1392-1407.

29.   Holmberg CI, Leppa S, Eriksson JE, Sistonen L. The phorbol ester 12-o-tetradecanoylphorbol 13-acetate enhances the heat-induced stress response. J Biol Chem 1997; 272: 67926798.

30.   DiDonato JA, Hayakawa M, Rothwarf DM, Zandi E, Karin M. A cytokine responsive IkappaB kinase that activates the transcription factor NF-kappaB. Nature 1997; 388: 548-554.

31.   Mann DL. Stress activated cytokines and the heart. Cytokine Growth Factor Rev 1996; 7: 341-354.

32.   Chandrasekar B, Colston JT, Freeman GL. Induction of proinflammatory cytokine and antioxidant enzyme gene expression following brief myocardial ishaemia. Clin Exp Immunol 1997; 108: 346-351.

33.   Herskowitz A, Choi S, Ansari AA, Wesselingh S. Cytokine mRNA expression in post-ischaemic reperfused myocardium. Am J Path 1995; 146: 419-428.

34.   Gurevitch J, Frolkis I, Yuhas Y et al. Tumour necrosis factor-alpha is released from the isolated heart undergoing ishcemia and reperfusion. J Am Coll Cardiol 1996; 28: 247-252.

35.   Golino P, Ragni M, Cirillo P et al. Effects of tissue factor induced by oxygen free radicals on coronary flow during reperfusion. Nature Medicine 1996; 2: 35-39.

36.   Latini R, Bianchi M, Correale E et al. Cytokines in acute myocardial infarction: selective increase in circulating tumor necrosis factor, its soluble receptor, and interleukin-1 receptor antagonist. J Cardiovasc Pharmacol 1994; 23: 1-6.

37.   Gurevitch J, Frolkis I, Yuhas Y et al. Anti-tumor necrosis factor-alpha improves myocaridial recovery after ischemia and reperfusion. J Am Coll Cardiol 1997; 15: 1554-1561.

38.   Feuerstein GZ, Wang X, Barone FC. Inflammatory gene expression in cerebral ischemia and trauma. Potential new therapeutic targets. Ann N Y Acad Sci 1997; 825: 179-193.

39.   Moriguchi T, Toyoshima F, Masuyama N, Hanafusa H, Gotoh Y, Nishida E. A novel SAPK/JNK kinase, MKK7, stimulated by TNF alpha and cellular stresses. EMBO J 1997; 16: 7045-7053.

40.   Beyaert R, Cuenda A, Vanden Berghe W et al. The p38/RK mitogen-activated protein kinase pathway regulates interleukin-6 synthesis response to tumor necrosis factor. EMBO J 1996; 15: 1914-1923.

41.   Brenner DA, O'Hara M, Angel P, Chojkier M, Karin M. Prolonged activation of jun and collagenase genes by tumour necrosis factor-α. Nature 1989; 337: 661-663.

42.   Sharma HS, Maulik N, Gho BCG, Das DK, Verdouw PD. Coordinated expression of heme oxygenase-1 and ubiquitin in the porcine heart subjected to ischemia and reperfuion. Mol Cell Biochem 1996; 157: 111-116.

43.   Watanabe N, Tsuji N, Akiyama S et al. Induction of heat shock protein 72 synthesis by endogenous tumor necrosis factor via enhancement of the heat shock element-binding activity of heat shock factor 1. Eur J Immunol 1997; 27: 2830-2834.

44.   Isoherranen K, Peltola V, Laurikainen L et al. Regulation of copper/zinc and manganese superoxide dismutase by UVB irradiation, oxidative stress and cytokines. J Photochem Photobiol 1997; 40: 288-293.

45.   Harris CA, Derbin KS, Hunte-McDonough B et al. Manganese superoxide dismutase is induced by IFN-gamma in multiple cell types. Synergistic induction by IFN-gamma and tumor necrosis factor or IL-1. J Immunol 1991; 147: 149-154.

46.   Thiagarajan RR, Winn RK, Harlan JM. The role of leukocyte and endothelial adhesion molecules in ischemia-reperfusion injury. Thromb Haemost 1997; 78: 310-4.

47.   Yamauchi-Takihara K, Ihara Y, Ogata A, Yoshizaki K, Azuma J, Kishimoto T. Hypoxic stress induces cardiac myocyte-derived interleukin-6. Circulation 1995; 91: 1520-1524.

48.   Haveman J, Geerdink AG, Rodermond HM. Cytokine production after whole body and localized hyperthermia. Int J Hyperthermia 1996; 12: 791-800.

49.   Beetz A, Messer G, Oppel T, van Beuningen D, Peter RU, Kind P. Induction of interleukin 6 by ionizing radiation in a human epithelial cell line: control by corticosteriods. Int J Radiat Biol 1997; 72: 33-43.

50.   Stephanou A, Isenberg DA, Akira S, Kishimoto T, Latchman DS. The nuclear factor interleukin-6 (NF-IL6) and signal transducer and activator of transciption-3 (STAT-3) signalling pathways co-operate to mediate the activation of the hsp90beta gene by interleukin-6 but have opposite effects on its inducibility by heat shock. Biochem J 1998; 15: 189-195.

51.   Pellegrini P, Berghella AM, Di Loreto S et al. Cytokine contribution to the repair processes and homeostatis recovery following anoxic insult: a possible IFN-gamma regulatory role in IL-1 beta neurotoxic action in physiological or damaged CNS. Neuroimmunomodulation 1996; 3: 213-218.

52.   Lu G, Beuerman RW, Zhao S et al. Tumor necrosis factor-alpha and interleukin-1 induce activation of MAP kinase and SAP kinase in human neuroma fibroblasts. Neurochem Int 1997; 4-5: 401-410.

53.   Karin M, Imbra RJ, Heguy A, Wong G. Interleukin-1 regulates human metallothionein gene expression. Mol Cell Biol 1985; 5: 2866-2869.

54.   Crosby AJ, Wahle KW, Duthie GG. Modulation of glutathione peroxidase activity in human vascular endothelial cells by fatty acids and the cytokine interleukin-1 beta. Biochim Biophys Acta 1996; 1303: 187-192.

55.   Massague J, Cheeifetz S, Laiho M, Ralph DA, Weis FMB, Zentella A. Transforming growth factor-b. Cancer Surveys 1992; 12: 81-103.

56.   Roberts AB, Roche NS, Winokur TS, Burmester JK, Sporn MB. Role of transforming growth factor-β in maintenance of function of cultured neonatal cardiac myocytes. J Clin Invest 1992; 90: 2056-2062.

57.   Falanga V, Qian SW, Danielpour D, Katz MH. Roberts AB, Sporn MB. Hypoxia upregulates the synthesis of TGF-β 1 by human dermal fibroblasts. J Invest Dermatol 1991; 97: 634-637.

58.   Flanders KC, Winokur TS, Holder MG, Sporn MB. Hyperthermia induces expression of transforming growth factor-βs in rat cardiac cells in vitro and in vivo. J Clin Invest 1993; 92: 404-410.

59.   Lefer AM, Tsao P, Aoki N, Palladino M. Mediation of cardioprotection by transforming growth factor-β. Science 1990; 249: 61-64.

60.   Kenny D, Coughlan MG, Pagel PS, Kampine JP, Warltier DC. Transforming growth factor-β_1 preserves endothelial function after multiple brief coronary artery occlusions and reperfusion. American Heart J 1994; 127: 1456-1461.

61.   Roberts AB, Sporn MB, Lefer AM, Cardioprotective actions of transforming growth factor-β. Trends Cardiovasc Med 1993; 3: 77-81.

62.   Kluge A, Zimmermann R, Mukel B, Verdouw P, Schaper J, Schaper W. Insulin-like growth factor II is an experimental stress inducible gene in a porcine model of brief coronary occlusions. Cardiovasc Res 1995; 29: 708-716.

63.   Lee WH, Seaman GM, Vannucci SJ. Coordinate IGF-I and IGFBP5 gene expression in perinatal rat brain after hypoxia-ischemia. J Cereb Blood Flow Metab 1996; 16: 227-236.

64.   Vogt AM, Htun P, Kluge A, Zimmermann R, Schaper W. Insulin-like growth factor-II delays myocardial infarction in experimental coronary artery occlusion. Cardiovasc Res 1997;33:469-477.

65.   Battler A, Hasdai D, Goldberg I et al. Exogenous insulin-like growth factor II enhances post-infarction regional myocardial function in swine. Eur Heart J 1995; 16: 1851-1859.

66.   Cuevas P, Carceller F, Lozano R, Crespo A, Zazo M, Gimenez-Gallego G. Protection of rat myocardium by mitogenic and non-mitogenic fibroblast growth factor during post-ischemic reperfusion. Growth Factors 1997; 15: 29-40.

67.   Williams AJ. The functions of two species of calcium channel in cardiac muscle excitation-contraction coupling. Eur Heart J 1997; 18: A27-A35.

68.   Kasai M, Ide T. Regulation of calcium release channel in sarcoplasmic reticulum. Ion Channels 1996; 4: 303-331.

69.   Kawakami M, Okabe E. Superoxide anion radical-triggered Ca^{2+} release from cardiac sarcoplasmic reticulum through ryanodine receptor Ca^{2+} channel. Mol Pharmacol 1998; 53: 497-503.

70.   Morris TE, Sulakhe PV. Sarcoplasmic reticulum Ca^{2+} pump dysfunction in rat cardiomyoctes briefly exposed to hydroxyl radicals. Free Radic Biol Med 1997; 22: 37-47.

71.   Grover AK, Samson SE, Misquitta CM. Sarco(endo)plasmic reticulum Ca^{2+} pump isoform SERCA3 is more resistant than SERCA2b to peroxide. Am J Physiol 1997; 273: C420-C425.

72.   Meldrum DR, Cleveland JC, Mitchell MB, Rowland RT, Banerjee A, Harken AH. Constructive priming of myocardium against ischemia-reperfusion injury. Shock 1996; 6: 238-242.

73.   Samouilidou EC, Karli JN, Levis GM, Darsinos JT. The sarcolemmal Ca^{2+}-ATPase of the ischemic-reperfused myocardium: protective effect of hypocalcemia on calmodulin-stimulated activity. Life Sci 1998; 62: 29-36.

74.   Frass O, Sharma HS, Knoll R et al. Enhanced gene expression of calcium regulatory proteins in stunned porcine myocardium. Cardiovasc Res 1993; 27: 2037-43.

75.   Linck B, Boknik P, Eschenhagen T et al. Messenger RNA expression and immunological quantification of phospholamban and $SR-Ca^{2+}$-ATPase in failing and nonfailing human hearts.Cardiovascular Research 1996; 31: 625-632.

76.   Flesch M, Schwinger RH, Schnabel P et al. Sarcoplasmic reticulum Ca^{2+} ATPase and phospholamban mRNA and protein levels in end-stage heart failure due to ischemic or dilated cardiomyopathy. J Mol Med 74: 321-332.

77.   Das DK, Maulik N, Moraru II. Gene expression in acute myocardial stress. Induction by hypoxia, ischemia, reperfusion, hyperthermia and oxidative stress. J Mol Cell Cardiol 1995; 27: 181-193.

78.   Fornace AJ, Alamo I, Hollander MC, Lamoreaux E. Ubiquitin mRNA is a major stress-induced transcript in mammalian cells. Nucleic Acids Res 1989 17: 1215-1230.

79.   Andres J, Sharma HS, Knoll R et al. Expression of heat shock proteins in the normal and stunned porcine myocardium. Cardiovascular Research 1993; 27: 1421-1429.

80.   Das DK, Moraru II, Maulik N, Engelman RM. Gene expression during myocardial adaptation to ischemia and reperfusion. Ann N Y Acad Sci 1994; 723: 292-307.

81.   Glatz JF, van Nieuwenhoven FA, Luiken JJ, Schaap FG, van der Vusse GJ. Role of membrane-associated and cytoplasmic fatty acid-binding proteins in cellular fatty acid metabolism. Prostaglandins Leukot Essent Fatty Acids 1997; 57: 373-378.

82.   Tanka T, Sohmiya K, Kawamura K. Is CD36 deficiency an etiology of hereditary hypertrophic cardiomyopathy? J Mol Cell Cardiol 1997; 29: 121-127.

83.   Miskin R, Reich E. Plasminogen activator: induction of synthesis by DNA damage. Cell 1980; 19: 217-224.

84.   Hubank M, Schatz DG. cDNA.RDA: a sensitive and flexible method for the identification of differentially expressed genes. In: S. M. Weissman (ed), Methods in Enzymology, London, Academic Press, 1998, in press.

85.   Brown AJH, Hutchings C, Burke JF, Mayne LV. Targeted Display, a new technique for the analysis of differential gene expression. In: S M Weissman (ed), Methods in Enzymology, London, Academic Press, 1998, in press.

7

The Heat Shock Response and Tissue Protection

R W Currie and J-C L Plumier

1. Introduction

The name of heat shock proteins (HSPs) comes from their initial discovery following heat shock treatment. In the early 1960s, Ferruccio Ritossa made the first observation that elevated temperature could trigger rapid and specific changes in chromosomal and metabolic activity of living organisms; new mRNA was synthesised within 2-3 minutes [1, 2]. During the 1970s several laboratories discovered that novel (heat shock) proteins were expressed in cells after brief elevation of temperature [3-5]. At about the same time it was also recognised that these changes in gene expression, induced by mild heat shock, were associated with a subsequent tolerance of cells [6] and organisms [7] to severe thermal injury. These pioneering studies in *Drosophila* cells [1-7] lead to discoveries of HSPs in all cells from bacteria to man [8], and of inducible and transient cellular protection in cells and organs as varied as heart, brain, kidney and retina, the subject of this chapter.

2. Heat Shock and HSP70

All living organisms respond to a wide variety stresses by synthesising HSPs. Individual HSPs are classified into several families according to their molecular weight (Table 1): the 110 kDa HSP family, the 90 kDa HSP family, the 70 kDa HSP family, the 60 kDa HSP family, the 27 kDa HSP family, and ubiquitin [9-11]. In mammals, the most interesting family of HSPs is the 70-kDa family. The 70 kDa family of HSPs consists of at least four members of specific molecular weight and subcellular location (Table 1). BiP (immunoglobulin-binding protein) or Grp78 (glucose regulated protein) has an apparent molecular weight of 78 kDa and is localised in the endoplasmic reticulum and golgi apparatus. HSP75 has an apparent molecular weight of 75 kDa and is localised in the mitochondria. HSC70 is the constitutive protein, with an apparent molecular weight of 73 kDa and has been referred to as HSP73 and HSC73 in rats and humans. In fact, HSC70, BiP and HSP75 are all constitutive proteins in most mammalian cells and after stress their expression is increased modestly compared to HSP70. HSP70 is at low or undetectable levels in many unstressed mammalian cells, is highly inducible, becoming the major product of protein synthesis after heat shock [12]. HSP70 has an apparent molecular weight of 71 kDa in rats and 72 kDa in humans, and has been referred to as (stress protein) SP71 and HSP71 in rats, and HSP72 in humans.

While HSP70 is normally at low constitutive levels in most cells, it is highly inducible and accumulates in cells to be a major component of total cellular protein. HSP70 mRNA is not detected normally in the heart and brain of rats. After heat shock treatment (42 °C for 15 minutes) of rats or rabbits mRNA for HSP70 is detectable in heart and brain within 30 minutes. Peak mRNA levels are present at 1.5 to 3 hours and return to near basal levels by 6 hours after heat shock treatment [13-15]. Synthesis of HSP70 protein follows a similar time course [12, 13, 16, 17]. HSP70 protein accumulates in heart and brain up to about 6 hours after heat shock treatment and it is then degraded slowly, still being easily detectable in the heart even two weeks after heat shock treatment [13, 17].

The role of HSPs during normal conditions and during stress is the subject of intense investigation. Recent evidence suggests that most HSPs can act as molecular chaperones and regulate protein folding and translocation [18-20]. Interestingly, specific expression of several HSPs has been shown to protect cells in culture against cell death induced by various means such as heat shock, oxidative injury, or cytokines [21-28]. In addition, it has been suggested that HSPs could also be protective to organs during and following pathological conditions such as ischaemia [29].

3. Heat Shock, HSP70 and Inducible Cellular Protection in Heart

Hyperthermic treatment of rats induces expression of HSP70 in the heart and all other tissues. This hyperthermic treatment followed by 24 hours of recovery, conditions the heart to respond differently after a second metabolic stress [29-33]. After 30 minutes of ischaemic injury, heat shocked hearts have a significantly improved recovery of contractility

Table 1. Classification, localisation and function of heat shock proteins

Protein	Intracellular localisation	Functions
Hsp110	nucleolus	- aids recovery of nucleolar transcription after stress
Hsp90	cytoplasm and nucleus	- regulates glucocorticoid receptor function - chaperones polypeptides to their cellular compartments
Hsc70	cytoplasm, nucleus and nucleolus	- uncoating of clathrin-coated vesicles - translocation of proteins across intracellular membranes - chaperones and folds nascent proteins - binds heat shock transcription factor
Hsp70 (inducible Hsp70, human Hsp72; rat Hsp71, SP71, P71)	cytoplasm, nucleus and nucleolus	- similar to Hsc70 - maintains solubility of cytosolic and nuclear proteins -facilitates the removal or folding of denatured proteins
BiP Grp78	endoplasmic reticulum	- facilitates assembly of monomeric proteins into larger macromolecules
Grp75 Mtp70	mitochondrial matrix	- similar to BiPin the mitochondria
Hsp60	mitochondria	- maintains polypeptides in unfolded state to facilitate translocation - accelerates proper folding/assembly
Hsp32 (heme oxygenase-1)	cytoplasm	- facilitates turnover of heme-containing protein
Hsp27 (murine Hsp25)	cytoplasm and nucleus	- helps folding of denatured protein - regulation of actin dynamics
ubiquitin	cytoplasm	- binds denatured polypeptides and targets them for degradation (recycling)

during reperfusion. Associated with this improved postischaemic contractile recovery is a reduction in creatine kinase release, indicative of less cellular injury. In addition, Yellon et al. [34] have shown a protective role for heat shock treatment in ischaemic and reperfused rabbit hearts. Donnelly et al. [35] have reported improved salvage of the ischaemic area of the myocardium in rats 24 hours post-heat shock. We showed that induction of the heat shock response (and 24 hours of recovery) in rabbits significantly reduced infarct size following *30 minutes* of coronary artery occlusion [14]. No reduction in infarct size was seen with 40 hours of recovery from the heat shock treatment or if the occlusion was extended to *45 minutes*. Similarly, Yellon et al. [36] reported no reduction in infarct size after a 45 minute coronary artery occlusion in rabbit hearts 24 hours post-heat shock. Together these results suggest that heat shock-induced myocardial protection is transient and has decayed by 40 hours post-heat shock and that the induced myocardial protection delays (but does not prevent) the onset of irreversible injury. For transplantation, the practical usefulness of heat shock treatment of rats is illustrated by the significantly improved recovery of isolated hearts from after 0 °C cardioplegic storage [37, 38]. In these studies myocardial protection is always associated with increased expression of the highly inducible HSP70. In fact, a direct correlation has been made between the level of HSP70 and the myocardial protection as measured by reduction in infarct size [39]. Recent studies have shown that a pharmacological approach to the induction of HSP70 expression provides myocardial protection that may be of clinical relevance [40-42].

4. HSP70 Transgenic Mice and Myocardial Protection

Myocardial protection has been reported in three strains of HSP70 transgenic mice. We examined the role of the human inducible HSP70 in transgenic mouse hearts [43]. Overexpression of the human HSP70 does not appear to affect normal protein synthesis or the stress response in transgenic mice compared with the non-transgenic mice. After 30 minutes of ischaemia, upon reperfusion, transgenic hearts versus non-transgenic hearts showed significantly improved recovery of contractile force, rate of contraction and rate of relaxation. Creatine kinase was released at a high level upon reperfusion from the non-transgenic hearts, but not the transgenic hearts. We concluded that high level constitutive expression of the human inducible HSP70 plays a direct role in the protection of the myocardium from ischaemia and reperfusion injury. Simultaneously, Dillmann's group [44, 45] showed similar findings of myocardial tolerance to ischaemic injury in hearts of transgenic mice overexpressing the rat inducible HSP70. In addition, Williams and his group [46] recently reported similar myocardial protection of energy metabolism in the hearts of transgenic mice overexpressing the human HSP70. Thus there is good evidence that HSP70 plays a role in myocardial protection.

5. Function of HSP70

Most evidence suggests that the HSP70 family of HSPs act as molecular chaperones (Figure 1) [47, 48]. In general, it is clear that HSPs are important in normal metabolism, and hence the relatively high constitutive level of most HSPs. HSC70 is thought to bind nascent protein to facilitate translocation and proper folding. BiP (immunoglobulin binding protein; GRP78, glucose regulated protein) binds and translocates nascent protein to the golgi apparatus. HSC70 and HSP60 are involved in importation of protein into the mitochondria and in facilitating folding of proteins to mature forms. Other HSPs such as ubiquitin, are important in targeting denatured proteins for degradation and hence the recycling of amino acids. One interesting function of the HSC70 is its interaction with the transcription factor, heat shock factor (HSF), under normal conditions [49, 50]. With stress the HSC70 and HSF separate allowing the HSF to trimerise, and bind to the heat shock elements on DNA to initiate transcription of new HSPs and particularly HSP70. HSP70 is thought to function at least in part, in a similar manner to HSC70 (Figure 1). HSP70 also seems to be important in unfolding of denatured protein and refolding proteins in mature form. Overall, these HSPs are important in maintaining solubility of proteins in the various compartments of the cell.

Recently, a novel pathway for HSP70 interaction has been identified. Elevated levels of HSP70 inhibit the signal transduction pathway leading to programmed cell death by preventing activation of the stress-activated protein kinase (SAPK)/Jun N-terminal kinase (JNK) [51]. In addition it was shown that elevated levels of abnormal proteins activated both the SAPK/JNK and p38 mitogen activated protein (MAP) kinase and that elevated levels of HSP70 blocked the activation of SAPK/JNK and p38 MAP kinase (Figure 2). Subsequently in another study HSP70 was found to be an up-stream blocker for the activation of SAPK/JNK, and also a down-stream blocker at the level of caspase-3 [52]. In fact it may be the chaperoning function of HSP70 that blocks the conversion of caspase-3. It was concluded that this pathway plays a major role in acquired cellular protection in mammalian cells.

6. Inducible Cellular Protection in the Brain

Heat shock treatment and ischaemia can induce cellular protection in other organs; the nervous system and the brain are particularly interesting. The first example of inducible protection in the nervous

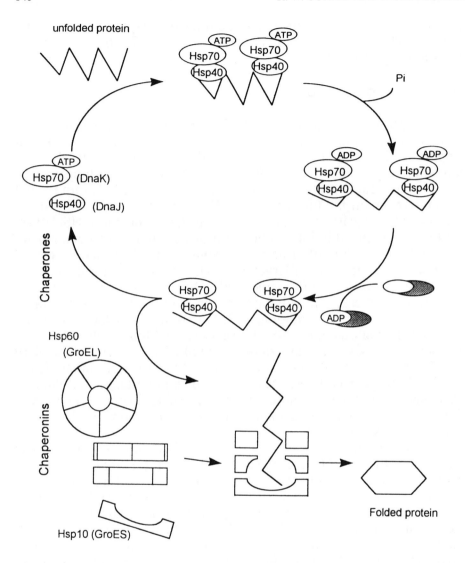

Figure 1. Chaperone activity of HSP70. The homolog proteins of *E. coli* are given in brackets [modified from 47, 48]. HSP70 and HSC70 are similar proteins and likely have similar function in chaperoning. The constitutive HSC70 is most abundant in unstressed cells.

system was that heat shock treatment of rats could prevent neuronal cell death in the retina caused by bright light [53]. Heat shock treatment was also able to protect cultured neurones from glutamate-induced excitotoxicity [54, 55]. In these experiments, heat shocked neurones were transiently protected at 3 hours and 24 hours but not at 48 hours after heat shock and were protected from a wide range of glutamate concentrations. Heat shock treatment also protects neurones in the brain from ischaemia. Hyperthermia 18 hours to 24 hours before a 5 to 7 minute episode of transient forebrain ischaemia significantly reduced neuronal cell death [56, 57]. In a similar fashion, a short episode of ischaemia protects neurones from a subsequent ischaemic insult of longer duration. Interestingly, in the brain this protection tends to be evident between 1 day and 7 days after the conditioning ischaemic insults [58-61] and elevated expression of HSP70 is usually associated with reduction of infarct size and/or less cell death. In recent experiments using transgenic mice overexpressing the human HSP70, infarct size in the brain was not reduced following 24 hours of ischaemic injury [62]. However, a less severe ischaemic injury might have revealed a smaller infarct compared to the non-transgenic controls. While infarct size was not different (suggesting that the mice were not anatomical or physiologically different), the HSP70 transgenic mice had no evidence of neuronal cell death in the hippocampus compared to significant cell loss in the hippocampus of the non-transgenic mice [62]. HSP70 may have protected the hippocampal neurones from ischaemia-induced cortical glutamate release and toxicity.

7. Other Possibilities

Following heat shock treatment, in addition to the increase in HSP70, there is also a significant increase in antioxidative enzyme activity [29, 63-66]. In these experiments catalase activity was elevated at 24 and 48 hours after heat shock and corresponded to the time of greatest protection of the myocardium from ischaemic injury [29, 63, 66]. In fact, inhibition of catalase with 3-amino-1,2,4-triazole 60 minutes before the onset of ischaemia disrupted the hyperthermia-induced cardioprotection. Thus catalase also appears to contribute to hyperthermia-induced cardioprotection. On the other hand, there is evidence that antioxidants are not involved in myocardial protection [67-69]. Interestingly, transgenic mice overexpressing HSP70 had no clear elevation in catalase activity [43, 44]. These findings suggest that there is more than one mechanism involved in adaptive myocardial protection.

Evidence is presented above that endogenous myocardial protection is attributable to at least two mechanisms, HSP70 and antioxidant enzymes. Another fascinating area of research is the rapidly acquired protection induced by classic ischaemic preconditioning [70].

While ischaemic preconditioning (i.e. a brief episode of ischaemia) induces a heat shock response, newly synthesised HSPs are not likely to be involved in this rapidly acquired protection. Recently, strong evidence has suggested that another heat shock protein, HSP27, contributes to cellular protection and possibly interacts with antioxidative enzymes.

8. HSP27 and Endogenous Cellular Protection

Other HSPs have been suggested to play a role in cellular resistance to injury. For example, transfection of the human HSP27 gene into NIH/3T3 cells, a fibroblast line, provides a measure of thermotolerance [21, 71, 72] and increases resistance to oxidative stress and tumour necrosis factor-α (TNF-α) induced cytotoxicity [73]. In fact, recent experiments have demonstrated that phosphorylated isoforms of HSP27 increased cell survival against lethal heat shock or cell death induced by hydrogen peroxide [74, 75].

Like HSP70, HSP27 acts as molecular chaperone and binds unfolded proteins during heat shock, preventing nonspecific aggregation of protein [76, 77]. In addition, it has been suggested that HSP27 might regulate actin filament organisation. In thermotolerant cells or in HSP27-transfected cells, heat shock-induced disassembly of actin filaments is prevented and recovery is more rapid. The protection of microfilament organisation appears to be a consequence of interaction between HSP27 and actin components, since HSP27 over-expression also protects against cytotoxicity induced by actin polymerisation inhibitor cytochalasin D [71, 72] and stabilises actin filaments during oxidative stress [75].

It has also been suggested that overexpression of human HSP27 reduces the intracellular generation of reactive oxygen species induced by treatment with TNF-α [27]. This protective effect of small HSPs was related to an increase in glutathione levels in three transfected cell lines and suggests that small HSPs regulate the level of antioxidative enzymes and thus the cellular susceptibility to oxidative stress. Another function for HSP27 might be regulation of mechanisms leading to apoptosis. HSP27 overexpression inhibited apoptosis induced by Fas/APO-1 receptor activation or treatment with staurosporine, a protein kinase C inhibitor [28]. Thus it seems that there may be more than a single role of HSP27 in cellular protection. Interestingly, the function of HSP27 might be regulated by its phosphorylation state. Under stressful conditions such as stimulation with hydrogen peroxide or cytokines, activation of the p38 MAP kinase causes increased phosphorylation of HSP27 (Figure 2) [78, 79]. HSP27 phosphorylation favours the shift of multimer HSP27 to monomer HSP27 [74].

9. HSP27 in the Heart and Brain

At the present time, the role of HSP27 in myocardial protection is not known. HSP27 is expressed in the rat heart after heat shock treatment [13] and after ischaemic injury [80]. Interestingly, treatment of rats with recombinant interleukin 1α-induced elevated levels of HSP27 mRNA and protein and elevated levels of antioxidative activities in hearts. Associated with these elevated levels of HSP27 and antioxidants was improved contractile recovery of the myocardium from ischaemic injury [81].

As in the heart, it is likely that inducible protection in the brain is due to more than one protein and one mechanism. As discussed above, HSP27 may play a role in chaperoning, regulating antioxidative enzymes and maintenance of actin filaments. HSP27 has been observed in Purkinje neurones of the cerebellum and in large neurones of the spinal cord in the developing mouse nervous system [82], but was not detected in the adult brain [83-85]. Recently, we have completed a study of the normal anatomical distribution of HSP27 in the rat central nervous system [86]. While no HSP27 was detected in the cerebral cortex, many lower neurones of the brain stem and spinal cord contained HSP27. Most general somatic efferent motor neurones of the oculomotor, trochlear and hypoglossal nuclei and spinal cord anterior horn were HSP27-positive as were special visceral efferent motor neurones of the trigeminal, facial, glossopharyngeal and vagal special visceral efferent motor nuclei. In contrast, general visceral efferent neurones of the dorsal motor nucleus of the vagus nerve contained few HSP27-positive neurones. The distribution of peripheral afferent projections occurred in distinct patterns of HSP27 immunoreactivity indicating that select subpopulations of afferent neurones express HSP27 constitutively [86]. In addition, we have also shown that HSP27 is highly induced in astrocytes of the cerebral cortex after status epilepticus [87], and cortical focal ischaemic injury [88]. In the latter study it was particularly evident that HSP27 was expressed in astrocytes throughout the injured cerebral cortex, beyond the focal injury. Interestingly, potassium chloride-induced cortical spreading depression, a known consequence of ischaemic injury in the brain, induced expression of HSP27 in astrocytes throughout the ipsilateral cortex [89]. Blocking of cortical spreading depression with MK-801, a N-methyl-D-aspartate receptor antagonist, suppressed the expression of HSP27 throughout the cortex, suggesting that glutamate release played a role in the expression of HSP27 in astrocytes. Most interesting is that brains conditioned with cortical spreading depression have a significant resistance to subsequent ischaemic injury [90, 91]. Together, these results suggest an intriguing possibility. HSP27 may protect astrocyte function during and after ischaemia and through astrocyte-neurone

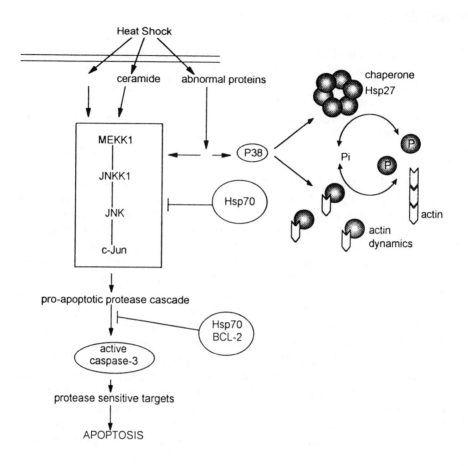

Figure 2. Stress activation of pathway leading to apoptosis. Elevated levels of HSP70 suppress activation of JNK/SAPK and caspase-3. Stress activation of p38 MAP kinase phosphorylates HSP27 and modulates its function [modified from 51, 52, 74, 78, 79].

interaction, improve neuronal survival. In fact such a protective effect of astrocytes on the survival of neurones after oxidative injury has been demonstrated in vitro in mixed astrocyte-neurone cultures [92]. It may be that HSP27 confers to astrocytes tolerance to ischaemic injury and that, by delaying astrocyte injury and the shut-down of astrocyte functions such as antioxidant activity or glutamate uptake, HSP27 contributes to the reduction of injurious stress affecting neurones.

10. Conclusions

Multi-cellular organisms have several ways of recovering from injury. One general strategy is to replace dead or injured cells by new functional cells. However, in the heart and in the brain, the functional cells, i.e., the myocytes and the neurones, are post-mitotic and cannot re-enter the cell cycle to replace lost cells. Thus, for post-mitotic cells, the ability to have rapid changes in gene expression seems to be of paramount importance for survival of the organism to changes in environmental conditions. Sub-lethal stresses such as ischaemia, oxidative injury, tissue trauma, fever, and of course hyperthermia, induce the expression of heat shock proteins, and in fact many other changes in gene expression. These responses to stress allow post-mitotic cells in the heart and brain to adjust and adapt to biochemical changes that may occur over decades.

In the heart and brain there are several strategies to protect against ischaemia. Firstly, there are cellular protective mechanisms within myocytes and neurones. These cellular protection mechanisms include synthesis of new proteins, such as HSPs, that will facilitate chaperoning, or increase the activity of constitutive enzymes, such as antioxidants. These changes reduce intracellular damage and contribute to a more rapid recovery of cellular function. Secondly, protective mechanisms are likely to include more than one role for some proteins. For example, HSP70 could act as a chaperone renaturing protein and as a regulator of pathways leading to apoptosis. Similarly, HSP27 could act as a chaperone, a regulator of antioxidative enzymes and play a role in actin dynamics. Thirdly, protective mechanisms could originate from co-operation of myocytes or neurones with other cells. For example, increased resistance of the small blood vessels to ischaemic injury or up-regulation of other supporting cells, could be an important component of such protective mechanisms. Most interesting is the possibility that HSP27 while upregulated in astrocytes and presumably playing a role in astrocyte function, protects neurones from ischaemic injury through cell-cell interactions.

Acknowledgements

This work is supported by the Heart and Stroke Foundation of New Brunswick. Dr Plumier was a recipient of a Research Traineeship Award from the Heart and Stroke Foundation of Canada, and currently is the recipient of a post-doctoral fellowship from the Cancer Research Society of Canada.

References

1.   Ritossa F. A new puffing pattern induced by temperature shock and DNP in Drosophila. Experientia 1962; 18: 571-573.

2.   Ritossa F. Discovery of the heat shock response. Cell Stress & Chaperones 1996; 1: 97-106.

3.   Tissieres A, Mitchell HK, Tracy U. Protein synthesis in salivary glands of Drosophila melanogaster. Relationship to chromosome puffs. J Mol Biol 1974; 84: 389-398.

4.   Lewis MJ, Helmsing P, Ashburner M. Parallel changes in puffing activity and patterns of protein synthesis in salivary glands of Drosophila. Proc Natl Acad Sci USA 1975; 72: 3604-3608.

5.   McKenzie S, Lindquist, Meselson M. Translation in vitro of Drosophila heat-shock messages. J Mol Biol 1977; 117: 279-283.

6.   Gerner EW, Schneider MJ. Induced thermal resistance in HeLa cells. Nature 1975; 256: 500-502.

7.   Mitchell HK, Moller G, Petersen NS, Lipps-Sarmento L. Specific protection from phenocopy induction by heat shock. Dev Genet 1979; 1: 181-192.

8.   Schlesinger ML, Ashburner M, Tissieres A. Heat shock: From bacteria to man. New York: Cold Spring Harbor Laboratory Press, 1982.

9.   Lindquist S. The heat-shock response. Annu Rev Biochem 1986; 55: 1151-1191.

10.   Welch WJ. The mammalian stress response: cell physiology and biochemistry of stress proteins. In: Morimoto RI, Tissieres A, Georgopoulos C (eds), Stress Proteins in Biology and Medicine. Cold Spring Harbor, Cold Spring Harbor Press, 1990: 223-278.

11.   Welch WJ. Mammalian stress response: cell physiology, structure/function of stress proteins, and implications for medicine and disease. Physiol Rev 1992; 72: 1063-1081.

12.   Currie RW, White FP. Trauma-induced protein in rat tissues: a physiological role for a "heat shock" protein? Science 1981; 214: 72-73.

13.   Currie RW, Tanguay RM. Analysis of rat heart RNA for transcripts for catalase and SP71 after in vivo hyperthermia. Biochem Cell Biol 1991; 67: 375-382.

14.   Currie RW, Tanguay RM, Kingma JG. Heat-shock response and limitation of tissue necrosis during occlusion/reperfusion in rabbit hearts. Circulation 1993; 87: 963-971.

15.   David J-C, Currie RW, Robertson HA. Expression and distribution of hsp71 and hsc73 messenger RNAs in rat brain following heat shock: effect of dizocilpine maleate. Neuroscience 1994; 62: 945-954.

16.   White FP, Currie RW. A mammalian response to trauma: the synthesis of a 71 kilodalton protein. In: Schlesinger ML, Ashburner M, Tissieres A (eds), Heat shock: From Bacteria to Man. New York: Cold Spring Harbor Laboratory Press, 1982: 379-386.

17.   Currie RW, White FP. Characterization of the synthesis and accumulation of a 71 kilodalton protein induced in rat tissues after hyperthermia. Can J Biochem Cell Biol 1983; 61:4 38-446.

18.   Pelham HRB. Speculations on the functions of the major heat shock and glucose regulated proteins. Cell 1986; 46: 959-961.

19.   Pelham HR. The retention signal for soluble proteins of the endoplasmic reticulum. Trends Biochem Sci 1990; 15: 483-486.

20.   Hartl FU. Molecular chaperones in cellular protein folding. Nature 1996; 381: 571-580.

21.   Landry J, Chretien P, Lambert H, Hickey E, Weber LA. Heat shock resistance conferred by expression of the human HSP27 gene in rodent cells. J Cell Biol 1989; 109: 7-15.

22.   Angelidis CE, Lazaridis I, Pagoulatos GN. Constitutive expression of heat-shock protein 70 in mammalian cells confers thermotolerance. Eur J Biochem 1991; 199: 35-39.

23.   Li GC, Li LG, Liu YK, Mak JY, Chen LL, Lee WM. Thermal response of rat fibroblasts stably transfected with the human 70-kDa heat shock protein-encoding gene. Proc Natl Acad Sci USA 1991; 88: 1681-1685.

24. Williams RS, Thomas JA, Fina M, German Z, Benjamin IJ. Human heat shock protein 70 (Hsp70) protects murine cells from injury during metabolic stress. J Clin Invest 1993; 92: 503-508.

25.   Mestril R, Chi S-H, Sayen MR, O'Reilly K, Dillmann WH. Expression of inducible stress protein 70 in rat heart myogenic cells confers protection against stimulated ischemia-induced injury. J Clin Invest 1994; 93: 759-767.

26.   Mehlen P, Preville X, Chareyron P, Briolay J, Klementz R, Arrigo A-P. Constitutive expression of human Hsp27, Drosophila Hsp27, or human alpha B-crystallin confer resistance to TNF-α and oxidative stress-induced cytotoxicity in stably transfected murine L929 fibroblasts. J Immunol 1995; 154: 363-374.

27.   Mehlen P, Kretz-Remy C, Preville X, Arrigo A-P. Human hsp27, Drosophila hsp27 and human (B-crystallin expression-mediated increase in glutathione is essential for the protective activity of these proteins against TNF-α-induced cell death. EMBO J 1996; 15: 2695-2706.

28.   Mehlen P, Schulze-Osthoff K, Arrigo A-P. Small stress proteins as novel regulators of apoptosis. Heat shock protein 27 blocks Fas/APO-1- and staurosporine-induced cell death. J Biol Chem 1996; 271: 16510-1614.

29.   Currie RW, Karmazyn M, Kloc M, Mailer K. Heat-shock response is associated with enhanced postischemic ventricular recovery. Circ Res 1988; 63: 543-549.

30.   Yellon DM, Latchman DS, Marber MS. Stress proteins and endogenous route to myocardial protection: fact or fiction? Cardiovasc Res 1993; 27: 158-161.

31.   Yellon DM, Marber MS. Hsp70 in myocardial ischaemia. Experientia 1994; 50: 1075-1084.

32.   Knowlton AA. The role of heat shock proteins in the heart. J Mol Cell Cardiol 1995; 27: 121-131.

33.   Mestril R, Dillmann WH. Heat shock proteins and protection against myocardial ischemia. J Mol Cell Cardiol 1995; 27: 45-52.

34.   Yellon DM, Latchman DS. Stress proteins and myocardial protection. J Mol Cell Cardiol 1992; 24: 113-124.

35.   Donnelly TJ, Sievers RE, Vissern FLJ, Welch WJ, Wolfe C. Heat shock protein induction in rat hearts. A role for improved myocardial salvation after ischemia and reperfusion? Circulation 1992; 85: 769-778.

36.   Yellon DM, Iliodromitis E, Latchman DS, Van Winkle DM, Downey JM, Williams FM, Williams TJ. Whole body heat stress fails to limit infarct size in the reperfused rabbit heart. Cardiovasc Res 1992; 26: 342-346.

37.   Amrani M, Corbett J, Boateng SY, Dunn MJ, Yacoub MH. Kinetics of induction and protective effect of heat-shock proteins after cardioplegic arrest. Ann Thorac Surg 1996; 61: 1407-1412.

38.   Zhang J, Furukawa RD, Fremes SE. The beneficial effects of heat-shock for prolonged hypothermic storage. J Surg Res 1996; 63: 314-319.

39.   Hutter MM, Sievers RE, Barbosa V, Wolfe CL. Heat-shock protein induction in rat hearts. A direct correlation between the amount of heat-shock protein induced and the degree of myocardial protection. Circulation 1994; 89: 355-360.

40.   Lee BS, Chen J, Angelidis C, Jurivich DA, Morimoto RI. Pharmacological modulation of heat shock factor 1 by antiinflammatory drugs results in protection against stress-induced cellular damage. Proc Natl Acad Sci USA 1995; 92: 7207-7211.

41.   Maulik N, Engelman RM, Wei Z et al. Drug-induced heat-shock preconditioning improves postischemic ventricular recovery after cardiopulmonary bypass. Circulation 1995; 92 (Suppl): II-381-II-388.

42.   Morris SD, Cumming DV, Latchman DS, Yellon DM. Specific induction of the 70-kD heat stress proteins by the tyrosine kinase inhibitor herbimycin-A protects rat neonatal cardiomyocytes. A new pharmacological route to stress protein expression? J Clin Invest 1996; 97: 706-712.

43.   Plumier J-CL, Ross BM, Currie RW et al. Transgenic mice expressing the human HSP70 have improved post-ischemic myocardial recovery. J Clin Invest 1995; 95: 1854-1860.

44.   Marber MS, Mestril R, Chi SH, Sayen MR, Yellon DM, Dillmann WH. Overexpression of the rat inducible 70-kD heat stress protein in a transgenic mouse increases the resistance of the heart to ischemic injury. J Clin Invest 1995; 95: 1446-1456.

45.   Hutter JJ, Mestril R, Tam EKW, Sieves RE, Dillmann WH, Wolfe CL. Overexpression of heat shock protein 72 in transgenic mice decreases infarct size in vivo. Circulation 1996; 94: 1408-1411.

46.   Radford NB, Fina M, Benjamin IJ et al. Cardioprotective effects of 70-kDa heat shock protein in transgenic mice. Proc Natl Acad Sci USA 1996; 93: 2339-2342.

47.   Morimoto RI, Tissieres A, Georgopoulos C. Progress and perspectives on the biology of heat shock proteins and molecular chaperones. In: Morimoto RI, Tissieres A, Georgopoulos C (eds), The Biology of Heat Shock Proteins and Molecular Chaperones. New York: Cold Spring Harbor Laboratory Press, 1994: 1-30.

48.   Hartman D, Gething M-J. Normal protein folding machinery. In: Feige U, Morimoto RI, Yahara I, Polla BS, (eds) Stress-inducible Responses. Basel: Birkhauser Verlag, 1996: 3-24.

49.   Morimoto RI, Sarge KD, Abravaya K. Transcriptional regulation of heat shock genes. J Biol Chem 1992; 267: 21987-21990.

50.   Morimoto RI. Cells in stress: transcriptional activation of heat shock genes. Science 1993; 259: 1409-1410.

51.   Gabai VL, Meriin AB, Mosser DD, et al. Hsp70 prevents activation of stress kinases. A novel pathway of cellular thermotolerance. J Biol Chem 1997; 272: 18033-18037.

52.   Mosser DD, Caron AW, Bourget L, Denis-Larose C, Massie B. Role of the human heat shock protein hsp70 in protection against stress-induced apoptosis. Mol Cell Biol 1997; 17: 5317-27.

53.   Barbe MF, Tytell M, Gower DJ, Welch WJ. Hyperthermia protects against light damage in the rat retina. Science 1988; 241: 1817-1820.

54.   Lowenstein DH, Chan PK, Miles MF. The stress protein response in cultured neurons: Characterization and evidence for a protective role in excitotoxicity. Neuron 1991; 7: 1053-1060.

55.   Rordorf G, Koroshetz WJ, Bonventre JV. Heat shock protects cultured neurons from glutamate toxicity. Neuron 1991; 7: 1043-1051.

56.   Kitagawa K, Matsumoto M, Tagaya M, et al. Hyperthermia-induced neuronal protection against ischemic injury in gerbils. J Cereb Blood Flow and Metab 1991; 11: 449-452.

57.   Chopp M, Chen H, Ho K.-L., et al. Transient hyperthermia protects against subsequent forebrain ischemic cell damage in the rat. Neurology 1989; 39: 1396-1398.

58.   Kato H, Lu Y, Araki T, Kogure K. Temporal profile of the effects of pretreatment with brief cerebral ischemia on the neuronal damage following secondary ischemic insult in the gerbil: cumulative damage and protective effects. Brain Res 1991; 553: 238-422.

59.   Kitagawa K, Matsumoto M, Kuwabara K, et al. Ischemic tolerance phenomenon detected in various brain regions. Brain Res. 1991; 561: 203-211.

60.   Liu Y, Kato H, Nakata N, Kogure K. Protection of rat hippocampus against ischemic neuronal damage by pretreatment with sublethal ischemia. Brain Res 1992; 586: 121-124.

61.   Chen J, Graham SH, Zhu RL, Simon RP. Stress proteins and tolerance to facal cerebral ischemia. J Cereb Blood Flow Metab 1996; 16: 566-577.

62.   Plumier J-CL, Krueger AM, Currie RW, Kontoyiannis D, Kollias G, Pagoulatos GN. Response of transgenic mice expressing the human 70-kDa heat shock protein to cerebral ischemia. Cell Stress Chaperones 1997; 2: 162-167.

63.   Karmazyn M, Mailer K, Currie RW. Acquisition and decay of heat-shock-enhanced postischemic ventricular recovery. Am J Physiol 1990; 259: H424-H431.

64.   Cornelussen R, Spiering W, Webers JH et al. Heat shock improves ischemic tolerance of hypertrophied rat hearts. Am J Physiol 1994; 267: H1941-H1947.

65.   Steare SE, Yellon DM. Increased endogenous catalase activity caused by heat stress does not protect the isolated rat heart against exogenous hydrogen peroxide. Cardiovasc Res 1994; 28: 1096-1101.

66.   Kingma JG, Simard D, Rouleau JR, Tanguay RM, Currie RW. Contribution of catalase to hyperthermia-mediated cardioprotection after ischemia-reperfusion in rabbits. Am J Physiol 1996; 270: H1165-H1171.

67. Wall SR, Fliss H, Korecky B. Role of catalase in myocardial protection against ischemia in heat shocked rats. Mol Cell Biochem 1993; 129: 187-194.

68. Auyeung Y, Sievers RE, Weng D, Barbosa V, Wolfe CL. Catalase inhibition with 3-amino-1,2,4-triazole does not abolish infarct size reduction in heat-shocked rats. Circulation 1995; 92: 3318-3322.

69. Rowland RT, Cleveland JC, Meng X, Ao L, Harken AH, Brown JM. A single endotoxin challenge induces delayed myocardial protection against infarction. J Surg Res 1996; 63: 193-198.

70.   Jennings RB, Steenbergen C Jr, Reimer KA. Myocardial ischemia and reperfusion. Monogr Pathol 1995; 37: 47-80.

71.   Lavoie JN, Gingras-Breton G, Tanguay RM, Landry J. Induction of Chinese hamster HSP27 gene expression in mouse cells confers resistance to heat shock. HSP27 stabilization of the microfilament organization. J Biol Chem 1993; 268: 3420-3429.

72.   Lavoie JN, Hickey E, Weber LA, Landry J. Modulation of actin microfilament dynamics and fluid phase pinocytosis by phosphorylation of heat shock protein 27. J Biol Chem 1993; 268: 24210-24214.

73.   Mehlen P, Kretz-Remy C, Briolay J, Fostan P, Mirault ME, Arrigo AP. Intracellular reactive oxygen species as apparent modulators of heat-shock protein 27 (hsp27) structural organization and phosphorylation in basal and tumour necrosis factor alpha-treated T47D human carcinoma cells. Biochem J 1995; 312: 67-75.

74.   Lavoie JN, Lambert H, Hickey E, Weber LA, Landry J. Modulation of cellular thermoresistance and actin filament stability accompanies phosphorylation-induced changes in the oligomeric structure of heat shock protein 27. Mol Cell Biol 1995; 15: 505-516.

75.   Huot J, Houle F, Spitz DR, Landry J. HSP27 phosphorylation-mediated resistance against actin fragmentation and cell death induced by oxidative stress. Cancer Res 1996; 56: 273-279.

76.   Jakob U, Gaestel M, Engel K, Buchner J. Small heat shock proteins are molecular chaperones. J Biol Chem 1993; 268: 1517-1520.

77.   Merck KB, Groenen PJ, Voorter CE, de Haard-Hoekman WA, Horwitz J, Bloemendal H, de Jong WW. Structural and functional similarities of bovine alpha-crystallin and mouse small heat-shock protein. A family of chaperones. J Biol Chem 1993; 268: 1046-1052.

78.   Huot J, Houle F, Marceau F, Landry J. Oxidative stress-induced actin reorganization mediated by the p38 mitogen-activated protein kinase/heat shock protein 27 pathway in vascular endothelial cells. Circ Res 1997; 80: 383-392.

79.   Guay J, Lambert H, Gingras-Breton G, Lavoie JN, Huot J, Landry J. Regulation of actin filament dynamics by p38 map kinase-mediated phosphorylation of heat shock protein 27. J Cell Sci 1997; 110: 357-368.

80.   Andres J, Sharma HS, Knoll R, Stahl J, Sassen LM, Verdouw PD, Schaper W. Expression of heat shock proteins in the normal and stunned porcine myocardium. Cardiovasc Res 1993; 27: 1421-1429. [erratum Cardiovasc Res 1993; 27: 1889.]

81.   Maulik N, Engelman RM, Wei Z, Lu D, Rousou JA, Das DK. Interleukin-1 alpha preconditioning reduces myocardial ischemia reperfusion injury. Circulation 1993; 88 (suppl): II-387-II-394.

82.   Gernold M, Knauf U, Gaestel M, Stahl J, Kloetzel PM. Development and tissue-specific distribution of mouse small heat shock protein hsp25. Dev Genet 1993; 14: 103-111.

83.   Klemenz R, Andres AC, Frohli E, Schafer R, Aoyama A. Expression of the murine small heat shock proteins hsp 25 and alpha B crystallin in the absence of stress. J Cell Biol 1993; 120: 639-645.

84.   Tanguay RM, Wu Y, Khandjian EW. Tissue-specific expression of heat shock proteins of the mouse in the absence of stress. Dev Genet 1993; 14: 112-118.

85.   Wilkinson JM, Pollard I. Immunohistochemical localisation of the 25 kDa heat shock protein in unstressed rats: Possible functional implications. Anat Rec 1993; 237: 453-457.

86.   Plumier J-CL, Hopkins DA, Robertson HA, Currie RW. Constitutive expression of the 27-kDa heat shock protein (Hsp27) in sensory and motor neurons of the rat nervous system. J Comp Neurol 1997; 384: 409-428.

87.   Plumier J-CL, Armstrong JN, Landry J, Babity JM, Robertson HA, Currie RW. Expression of the 27,000 mol wt heat shock protein following kainic acid-induced status epilepticus in the rat. Neuroscience 1996; 75: 849-856.

88.   Plumier J-CL, Armstrong JN, Wood NI et al. Differential expression of c-fos, hsp70 and hsp27 after photothrombotic injury in the rat brain. Mol Brain Res 1997; 45: 239-246.

89.   Plumier J-CL, David J-C, Robertson HA, Currie RW. Cortical application of potassium chloride induces the low molecular weight heat shock protein (Hsp27) in astrocytes. J Cereb Blood Flow Metab 1997; 17: 781-790.

90.   Kobayashi S, Harris VA, Welsh FA. Spreading depression induces tolerance of cortical neurons to ischemia in rat brain. J Cereb Blood Flow Metab 1995; 15: 721-727.

91.   Matsushima K, Hogan MJ, Hakim AM. Cortical spreading depression protects against subsequent focal cerebral ischemia in rats. J Cereb Blood Flow Metab 1996; 16: 221-226.

92.   Desagher S, Glowinski J, Premont J. Astrocytes protect neurons from hydrogen peroxide toxicity. J Neuroscience 1996; 16: 2553-2562.

8

Antioxidant Defences in Myocardial Adaptation: Role of Manganese Superoxide Dismutase in Delayed Preconditioning

N Yamashita, T Kuzuya and M Hori

1. Introduction

Increasing evidence suggests that myocardium becomes tolerant to ischaemic injury after exposure to sublethal cellular stresses, such as ischaemia [1], heat stress [2], endotoxin [3], and cytokines [4,5]. The classic preconditioning phenomenon, in which brief, nonlethal ischaemia, rapidly increases the tolerance of the heart to subsequent lethal ischaemia, has been observed in experimental models [1] and in patients [6,7]. The mechanism of classic preconditioning has been examined with regard to adrenergic stimulation [8,9], the ATP-sensitive K^+ channel [10, 11], protein kinase C activation [12, 13], and adenosine metabolism [12, 14]. However, the signal transduction system and the final effector of the protection are still a matter of discussion. Recently, we [15] and another group [16] found that the protective effect disappeared 3 hours after classic preconditioning and reappeared 24 hours after the initial nonlethal ischaemia. This late effect of ischaemic preconditioning was named the second window of protection [16]. Although de novo protein synthesis is not involved in the mechanism of classic preconditioning [17], the time course of the second window suggests that the synthesis of intrinsic proteins after the initial ischaemic stress is involved in the mechanism of the late phase effect. Among them, the induction of heat shock proteins was reported to have a parallel with the acquisition of tolerance to ischemia-reperfusion injury [18, 19].

We also found that an intrinsic radical scavenger, manganese superoxide dismutase (Mn-SOD), was induced in the preconditioned myocardium [20, 21] coincident with the acquisition of tolerance to ischaemia-reperfusion injury in dog hearts [15]. Oxygen radicals are produced in ischaemia-reperfused heart tissue and cause myocardial injury by means of lipid peroxidation of the sarcolemmal membrane [22]. Mn-SOD is located in mitochondria and is thought to play a major role in "front line" scavenging of superoxide generated by the electron transport system. Therefore, the induction of Mn-SOD by ischaemic preconditioning has a rationale in the cardioprotection against oxidative stress imposed by ischaemia-reperfusion. In this review, we focus on the antioxidant defences in myocardial adaptation, especially on the role of Mn-SOD in delayed cardioprotection (second window of protection).

2. Sublethal Ischaemia-induced Cardioprotection

The induction and activation of Mn-SOD thus could be the mechanism producing the protective effect of the second window of protection. To examine this hypothesis, we measured the Mn-SOD content in canine myocardium after preconditioning with four 5 minute left anterior descending coronary artery (LAD) occlusions [20]. Mn-SOD protein was measured by enzyme-linked immunosorbent assay soon after and at 3, 6, 12 and 24 hours after ischaemic preconditioning. Mn-SOD content in the subendocardium increased gradually with a peak (40% increase) observed 24 hours after sublethal ischaemia. At this peak point, myocardial Mn-SOD activity, measured simultaneously by the nitroblue tetrazolium method, was also increased by about 60 % of normal control. We did not detect any differences in other antioxidant enzyme activities, including Cu,Zn-SOD, catalase, and glutathione peroxidase.

Next we demonstrated that this ischaemic preconditioning protocol resulted in a delayed protective response against myocardial necrosis after subsequent prolonged ischaemia in the dog [15]. We examined the effect of repeated brief ischaemia on the limitaton of infarct size. Immediately after or at 3, 12, and 24 hours after four 5 minute occlusions of LAD, dogs were subjected to 90 minutes LAD occlusion followed by 5 hours reperfusion. When the second ischaemic episode was applied immediately after the sublethal ischaemia, the percentage of risk area infarcted was markedly decreased to 14% compared with 42% in the control, the classic preconditioning effect. However, statistically-significant limitation of myocardial infarction was not observed when the time interval between sublethal and sustained ischaemia was 3 or 12 hours. Interestingly, the infarct-limiting effect was observed again 24 hours after ischaemic preconditioning. The time course of the reappearance of tolerance to

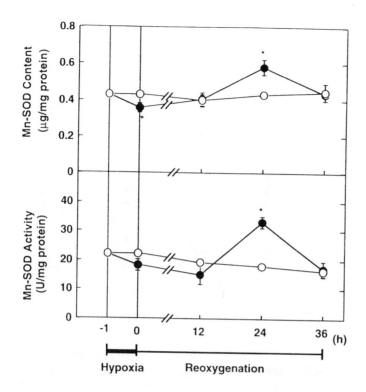

Figure 1. Mn-SOD content and activity in cultured cardiac myocytes after hypoxic preconditioning. The SOD activity in cultured myocytes without (open circles) or with (closed circles) hypoxic preconditioning was determined by the nitroblue tetrazolium method. The Mn-SOD content in the supernatant was determined by enzyme-linked immunosorbent assay. Eight batches of myocyte culture were examined for each data point. Means ± S.E.M. * $p < 0.05$. Reproduced from J Clin Invest 1994; 94: 2193-2199 by permission of The Rockefeller University Press.

ischaemia-reperfusion injury was identical with that of Mn-SOD induction in the preconditioned myocardium.

To investigate the role of enhanced Mn-SOD activity in protection against ischaemia-reperfusion injury directly, we examined whether the preconditioning phenomenon could be mimicked in cultured rat myocytes by exposing them to hypoxia (7 mmHg oxygen tension for 60 minutes) and reoxygenation (143 mmHg oxygen tension) before exposure to a subsequent sustained hypoxia-reoxygenation protocol [23]. Figure 1 shows the change in cardiac Mn-SOD content and activity after exposure to hypoxia in cultured cardiac myocytes. In control cells, which were subjected to normoxia instead of hypoxia for the first hour, Mn-SOD content and activity either did not change or showed a slight decrease

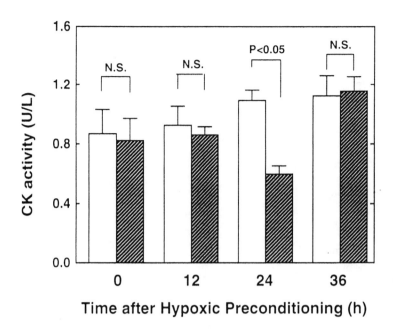

Figure 2. Creatine kinase (CK) release from myocytes after hypoxia-reoxygenation.CK release after second reoxygenation for 1 hour following sustained hypoxia for 3 hours. Control cells were exposed to normoxic conditions instead of hypoxic preconditioning for 1 hour. Open columns, control myocytes; hatched columns, hypoxic preconditioned myocytes. N.S., Not significant. Reprinted from J Clin Invest 1994; 94: 2193-2199 by permission of the Rockefeller University Press.

during the following 36 hours. On the other hand, in the cells exposed to hypoxia, both the activity and the content of Mn-SOD increased markedly at 24 hours after reoxygenation from hypoxia. Mn-SOD induction was regulated at the transcriptional level, because Mn-SOD mRNA after hypoxia-reoxygenation increased and reached its peak at 30 minutes after reoxygenation.

Next we examined creatine kinase (CK) release from myocyte cultures after exposure to prolonged hypoxia for 3 hours followed by reoxygenation (Figure 2). In the control experiments in which cells were exposed to normoxia instead of hypoxia for the first hour, CK release after the second hypoxia remained constant up to 36 hours. However, in the cells exposed to 1 hour of hypoxia, CK release from myocyte cultures was markedly reduced when the second hypoxia was applied 24 hours after the first hypoxia compared with the cells without simulated preconditioning. The time course of this increase in myocardial tolerance to hypoxia of these myocytes after exposure to a brief preceding hypoxia was apparently similar to that of Mn-SOD induction.

To examine the cause-and-effect relationship between Mn-SOD induction and tolerence to hypoxia, we attempted to block Mn-SOD induction after hypoxia using antisense oligodeoxyribonucleotides to Mn-SOD mRNA. After confirming that antisense to Mn-SOD mRNA inhibited the induction of Mn-SOD protein, we examined the effect of antisense on CK release from myocytes after exposure to prolonged hypoxia. CK release from myocyte cultures was attenuated by 51% when the cells were exposed to a preceding brief hypoxia compared to that from cells without such exposure. However, antisense to Mn-SOD abolished the expected decrease in CK release from myocytes with hypoxic preconditioning. Sense oligodeoxyribonucleotides did not change CK release from preconditioned myocytes. These results indicate that Mn-SOD induction in cardiac myocytes after exposure to brief hypoxia is the mechanism for acquisition of tolerance to lethal hypoxia in cardiac myocytes.

3. Sublethal Heat Stress-induced Cardioprotection

3.1. In Vivo Studies

Whole-body hyperthermia also induces tolerance of the heart to ischaemia-reperfusion injury 24 - 48 hours after hyperthermia [2, 16, 24, 25]. This phenomenon is related to the amount of 72 kDa heat-shock protein (HSP72; inducible form) that is induced by heat shock [18, 19]. Das et al. [26] reported that mammalian hearts subjected to heat shock increase expression of Mn-SOD mRNA. Heat shock also enhances SOD activity in the pig heart [27]. Therefore, we investigated whether heat shock-induced cardioprotection is correlated with the induction of HSP72 or Mn-SOD, by comparing the time course of the induction of HSP72 and Mn-SOD after heat stress and of the development of tolerance to ischaemia-reperfusion injury in rats [28].

Whole-body hyperthermia was induced in anaesthetised rats by placing them in a temperature-controlled water bath (42 °C for 15 min). After recovery at room temperature, ischaemia was induced by occlusion of the left coronary artery (LCA) in vivo for 20 minutes followed by reperfusion for 48 hours and infarct size assessment. Both the incidence of ventricular fibrillation (VF) during ischaemia and the size of myocardial infarction were attenuated when the LCA was occluded 30 minutes after hyperthermia (Figure 3). The reduction in infarct size and VF incidence during LCA occlusion returned to control level 24 hours after hyperthermia. However, tolerance reappeared after 36 hours. The peak protection was observed 72 hours after hyperthermia. These results indicated that whole-body hyperthermia increased myocardial tolerance to ischaemia-reperfusion injury biphasically, similar to ischaemic preconditioning.

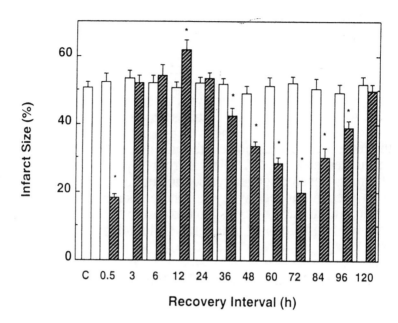

Figure 3. The effects of hyperthermic treatment on myocardial infarct size. After recovery from whole-body hyperthermia (42 °C for 15 minutes) ischaemia was induced by coronary occlusion for 20 minutes followed by reperfusion for 48 hours. Open columns: sham control rats with normothermia; hatched columns: hyperthermic treated rats. * p<0.05 vs sham control group.

We next examined the time courses of the induction of HSP72 and Mn-SOD after whole-body hyperthermia. Figure 4 shows the time course of HSP72 expression in heart tissue after whole-body hyperthermia, examined by Westhern blot analysis. HSP72 content was not altered at 30 mniutes after hyperthermia but showed a marked increase at 3 hours after hyperthermia. The HSP72 content remained elevated from 3-72 hours and then began to decrease, returning to the sham control value by 120 hours after hyperthermia. In the sham control group with normothermia, induction of HSP72 was not observed. These results suggested that HSP72 is induced after hyperthermia in vivo. However, the continuous expression of HSP72 can not account for the biphasic pattern of tolerance to ischaemia-reperfusion injury acquired following hyperthermia. Figure 5 shows the time course of Mn-SOD expression in heart tissue after whole-body hyperthermia examined by enzyme-linked immunosorbent assay. In the sham group with normothermia, Mn-SOD content did not change during the experimental time course In hyperthermia group, Mn-SOD content did not increase within the first 24 hours after hyperthermia. However, the content of Mn-SOD increased 48-72 hours after whole-body hyperthermia. These results indicate that the time course of the

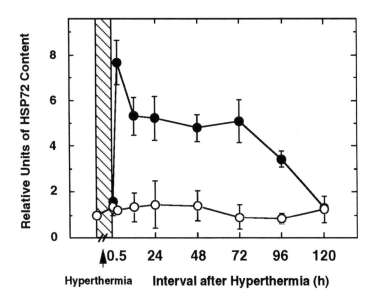

Figure 4. Densitometric assessment of Western blots of HSP72 content in heart tissue. Each data point represents the average of measurements in 3 tissue specimens. Closed circles: hyperthermic treated rats; open circles: sham control group. The relative levels of HSP72 were determined using optical densitometry and were normalised to the band of HSP72 detected in control rats. Modified from J Mol Cell cardiol 1997; 29: 1815-1821 with permission of Academic Press Ltd.

delayed cardioprotection induced by whole-body hyperthermia is in parallel with that of Mn-SOD induction, but not HSP72 induction.

3.2. In Vitro Studies

To examine whether heat shock-associated induction of Mn-SOD or HSP72 plays an important role in the induction of myocardial tolerance to ischaemia-reperfusion injury, we employed a heat shock model in cardiac myocytes in vitro [29]. We applied heat shock to myocytes and examined the induction of Mn-SOD protein and mRNA together with HSP72. Mn-SOD mRNA exhibited transient expression that peaked at 30 minutes after heat shock for 1 hour at 42 °C. HSP72 mRNA expression probed with a polymerase chain reaction (PCR) fragment of mouse cDNA was also increased dramatically at 30 minutes after heat shock. Twenty four hours after the cardiac myocytes were exposed to heat shock, HSP72 content of the cells was measured by Western blotting. Compared with untreated

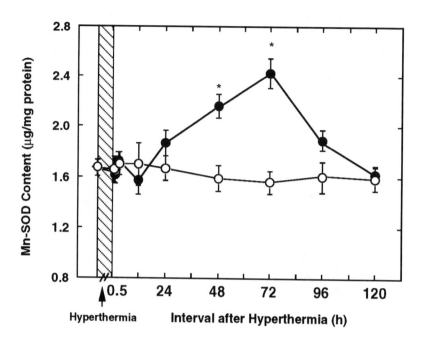

Figure 5. Mn-SOD content in myocardial tissue. Time course of the Mn-SOD content in myocardial tissue of hyperthermic (42 °C for 15 min) and sham control groups was determined by enzyme-linked immunosorbent assay. At least 4 rats were examined for each data point. Means ± S.E.M. * $p<0.05$ vs corresponding sham control groups.

cells, the HSP72 content had increased significantly in the heat-shocked cells. Similarly, the Mn-SOD content increased significantly 24 h after the heat shock, reaching about 140% of the level in untreated control cells.

As we had confirmed that heat shock induces both Mn-SOD and HSP72 in myocardial cells, we examined whether induction of these proteins plays any role in the acquisition of tolerance to hypoxia after heat shock. Heat shock for 1 hour at 42 °C increased the tolerance of myocytes to hypoxia, and reduced CK release by 60% compared with control cells without heat shock. Antisense to Mn-SOD inhibited Mn-SOD induction after heat shock (Figure 6) and also attenuated significantly this decrease in CK release (Figure 7). As the antisense oligodeoxyribonucleotide specifically inhibited Mn-SOD induction, HSP72 content level after heat shock was not reduced by the oligonucleotides.

These results indicate that Mn-SOD is induced after heat shock together with HSP72 and the former plays a pivotal role in the acquisition of tolerance to simulated ischaemia after heat shock. The role of Mn-SOD

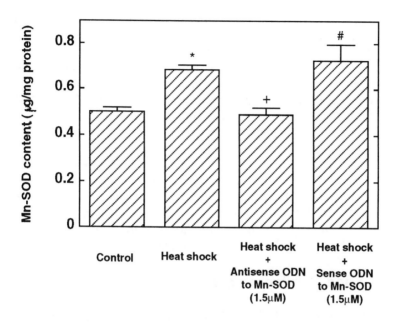

Figure 6. Induction of Mn-SOD protein 24 hours after heat shock (1 hour at 42 °C) in cardiomyocytes. Mn-SOD content was determined by enzyme-linked immunosorbent assay. Antisense or sense oligodeoxyribonucleotides (ODN) to Mn-SOD were added to the cultures from 18 hours before until 24 hours after heat shock. Data represent the mean ± SEM of six batches of cultured myocytes. * p<0.05 vs control, + p<0.05 vs heat shock, # p<0.05 vs heat shock + antisense ODN. Reproduced from J Mol Cell Cardiol 1997; 29: 1805-1813 with permission of Academic Press Ltd.

in cardioprotection might be independent from the induction of HSP72 because inhibition of Mn-SOD alone by antisense oligodeoxyribonucleotides abolished the tolerance hypoxia-reoxygenation injury. Because we could not design an effective oligonucleotide to inhibit HSP72 induction after heat shock, the experiment to suppress HSP72 alone was not performed. Although the inhibition of Mn-SOD alone specifically abolished the tolerance in our isolated cell model, the induction of HSPs, which acts as a molecular chaperones, might be involved in the adaptive mechanism. Beckmann et al. [30] have shown that members of the HSP70 family bind transiently to nascent proteins and act as intracellular chaperones, helping to stabilise these proteins until they achieve their final conformation. Voos et al. [31] have suggested that the constitutively expressed HSP70 in yeast cells may be an unfoldase that facilitates protein transport through the membranes of the endoplasmic reticulum and mitochondria. The induced HSP72 may have both chaperone functions and may help refold partially denatured proteins after stress. Thus, induction of HSP72 may promote the maturation of Mn-SOD. In a preliminary study, overexpression of HSP70 in rat hearts is reported to induce cardioprotection against ischaemia-reperfusion injury and is associated with increased levels of myocardial Mn-SOD content [32]. However, it remains to be determined if HSP72 and Mn-SOD are co-operative or interacting factors in acquired ischaemic tolerance.

It was shown that endogenous catalase activity in myocardium was also increased after heat stress and could protect heart against ischaemia-reperfusion injury [2, 25, 33, 34]. In these studies, we did not examine the catalase activity in myocytes or myocardium. It is conceivable, however, that a heat shock-induced increase in endogenous catalase activity in the cardiac myocytes could facilitate or enhance the detoxification of the superoxide in mitochondria and thus result in reduced injury to the cells during the process of ischaemia-reperfusion.

4. Exercise and Cardioprotection

Exercise is also assumed to be a physical stress that induces tolerance of the heart to ischaemia-reperfusion injury. Therefore, we set up an exercise training model of rats to examine if exercise reduces ischaemia-reperfusion injury through the induction of Mn-SOD [35]. Wistar rats were subjected to treadmill exercise, running at a rate of 25-30 m per minute for 25-30 minutes. At intervals from 30 minutes to 72 hours after exercise, the animals were anaesthetised and the LCA was occluded in vivo for 20 minutes followed by reperfusion for 48 hours. Rats that underwent LCA occlusion 30 minutes after exercise demonstrated a decrease in infarct size and reduced VF incidence during ischaemia compared with controls. Infarct size and the VF incidence during ischaemia retured to control values 24 hours after exercise. The tolerance reappeared from 36 hours after exercise and the peak protection was observed at 48 hours after exercise. These results indicate that treadmill exercise induced tolerance of the heart to ischaemia-reperfusion injury in a biphasic pattern, similar to the ischemic preconditioning and whole-body hyperthermia. We examined Mn-SOD content in myocardial tissue after treadmill exercise by enzyme-linked immunosorbent assay. Mn-SOD content in myocardial tissue did not increase 30 minutes after exercise. However, the content of Mn-SOD increased significantly 48 hours after treadmill exercise coincident with the acquisition of ischaemic tolerance. These results indicate that not only ischaemic preconditioning, but also physical stresses, such as hyperthermia and exercise induce the tolerance of the heart to ischaemia-reperfusion injury in a biphasic pattern. The induction of Mn-SOD in myocardium plays an important role in the delayed cardioprotection induced by these physical stresses.

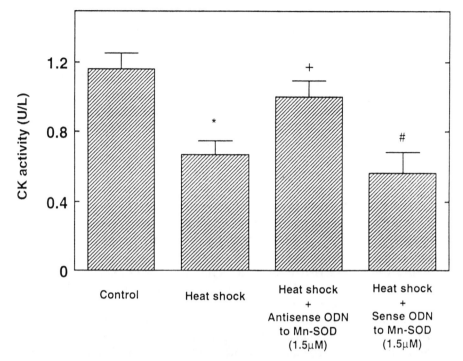

Figure 7. Effect of heat shock (1 hour at 42 °C) on myocardial cell injury after hypoxia-reoxygenation in cultured cardiomyocytes. Cell injury was assessed by measuring creatine kinase (CK) activity in the culture medium. Antisense or sense oligodeoxyribonucleotides (ODN) were added to myocytes from 18 h before to 24 h after heat shock. Data represent the mean ± SEM of six batches of cultured myocytes. * p<0.05 vs control, + p<0.05 vs heat shock, # p<0.05 vs heat shock + antisense ODN. Reproduced from J Mol Cell Cardiol 1997; 29: 1805-1813 with permission of Academic Press Ltd.

5. Production of Oxygen Free Radicals and Biphasic Cardioprotection

In ischaemic preconditioning, cardioprotection during the early phase may be mediated by the oxygen free radicals produced during preconditioning in rabbit in vivo [36-38] and rat heart in vitro [39]. The production of free radicals during ischaemic preconditioning is also involved in the mechanism of tolerance in the second window of protection against myocardial stunning in conscious pigs [40] (see chapter 2) and against myocardial infarction in rats [41]. Induction of Mn-SOD has been demonstrated in eukaryotes in conditions that favour the production of free radicals such as superoxide anion [42]. The induction of Mn-SOD by tumour necrosis factor was shown to be mediated by oxygen free radicals

(43). Therefore, we examined if an oxygen free radical mediated mechanism is involved in the acquisition of tolerance to ischaemia-reperfusion injury and in the induction of Mn-SOD after whole-body hyperthermia and exercise.

As described earlier, whole-body hyperthermia (42 °C for 15 minutes) reduced the incidence of VF during ischaemia and the size of myocardial infarction at 30 minutes (early-phase) and 72 hours (late-phase) after hyperthermia. Administration of N-2-mercaptopropionyl glycine (MPG), an antioxidant and a free radical scavenger, prior to hyperthermia abolished both the early- and late-phase cardioprotection and the corresponding late increase in Mn-SOD content. Treatment with MPG during exercise also abolished both the early-phase (30 minutes after exercise) and late-phase (48 hours after exercise) cardioprotection and the corresponding late increase in Mn-SOD content. In our preliminary study we measured Mn-SOD activity following ischaemic preconditioning in rat myocardium. Mn-SOD increased in a biphasic pattern similar to the ischaemic tolerance. However, Mn-SOD content increased only during the late phase. Administration of MPG during ischaemic preconditioning also abolished the early phase and late phase cardioprotection and the corresponding increase in Mn-SOD activity and late increase in Mn-SOD content. Similarly Zhou et al. also reported that in isolated rat myocytes, Mn-SOD activity increased after preconditioning with repetitive brief anoxia in a biphasic patter, similar to the pattern of anoxic tolerance. Administration of exogenous SOD during anoxic preconditioning abolished the late cytoprotection and the late increase in Mn-SOD activity [44]. These results indicate that free radical production in myocardial tissue may serve as a signal transduction pathway, which lead to the cardioprotection in a biphasic manner. The activation and/or induction of Mn-SOD, which is mediated by free radical production during ischaemic preconditioning, hyperthermia or exercise, is important in the acquisition of late-phase cardioprotection against ischaemia-reperfusion injury in rats.

6. Conclusion

In this chapter, we have reviewed how myocardium can acquire tolerance to ischaemia-reperfusion injury after exposure to physical stresses such as ischaemic preconditioning, whole-body hyperthermia, and exercise. We suggest that the production of oxygen free radicals in myocardial tissue is involved in the signal transduction pathways which link physical stresses to the acquisition of ischaemic tolerance in a biphasic manner. Although rescue proteins, including Mn-SOD and HSP72, were induced in the myocardium after these physical stresses, the induction of Mn-SOD correlate better with the delayed cardioprotection (second window of protection). Further studies should be done regarding the interaction or the sequence of action of these proteins and the signal transduction mechanism by which external stresses lead to the induction of the rescue proteins.

Acknowledgements

We thank Dr Shiro Hoshida for suggestions and help in the preparation of this manuscript. The studies described here were supported in part by a research grant from the Ministries of Education, Science and Culture awarded to Dr Kuzuya.

References

1.   Murry CE, Jennings RB, Reimer KA. Preconditioning with ischemia: a delay of lethal cell injury in ischemic myocardium. Circulation 1986; 74: 1124-1136.

2.   Currie RW, Karmazyn M, Kloc M, Mailer K. Heat-shock response is associated with enhanced postischemic ventricular recovery. Circ Res 1988; 63: 543-549.

3.   Brown JM, Grosso MA, Terada LS, et al. Endotoxin pretreatment increases endogenous myocardial catalase activity and decreases ischemia-reperfusion injury of isolated rat hearts. Proc Natl Acad Sci USA 1989; 86: 2516-2520.

4.   Brown JM, White CW, Terada LS, et al. Interleukin 1 pretreatment decreases ischemia/reperfusion injury. Proc Natl Acad Sci USA 1990; 87: 5026-5030.

5.   Eddy LJ, Goeddel DV, Wong GHW. Tumor necrosis factor-α pretreatment is protective in a rat model of myocardial ischemia-reperfusion injury. Biochem Biophys Res Commun 1992; 184: 1056-1059.

6.   Nakagawa Y, Ito H, Kitakaza M, et al. Effect of angina pectoris on myocardial protection in patients with reperfused anterior wall myocardial infarction: retrospective clinical evidence of "preconditioning". J Am Coll Cardiol 1995; 25: 1076-1083.

7.   Ottani F, Galvani M, Ferrini D, et al. Prodromal angina limits infarct size. A role for ischemic preconditioning. Circulation 1995; 91: 291-297.

8.   Banerjee A, Locke-Winter C, Rogers KB, et al. Preconditioning against myocardial dysfunction after ischemia and reperfusion by an α_1-adrenergic mechanism. Circ Res 1993; 73: 656-670.

9.   Kitakaze M, Hori M, Morioka T, et al. Alpha$_1$-adrenoceptor activation mediates the infarct size-limiting effect of ischemic preconditioning through augmentation of 5'-nucleotidase activity. J Clin Invest 1994; 93: 2197-2205.

10.   Gross GJ, Auchampach JA. Blockade of ATP-sensitive potassium channels prevents myocardial preconditioning in dogs. Circ Res 1992; 70: 223-233.

11.   Yao Z, Gross GJ. A comparison of adenosine-induced cardioprotection and ischemic preconditioning in dogs: efficacy, time course, and role of K_{ATP} channels. Circulation 1994; 89: 1229-1236.

12.   Downey JM, Cohen MV, Ytrehus K, Liu Y. Cellular mechanisms in ischemic preconditioning: the role of adenosine and protein kinase C. Ann NY Acad Sci 1994; 723: 82-98.

13.   Speechly-Dick ME, Mocanu MM, Yellon DM. Protein kinase C: its role in ischemic preconditioning in the rat. Circ Res 1994; 75: 586-590.

14.   Liu GS, Thornton J, Van Winkle DM, Stanley AW, Olsson RA, Downey JM. Protection against infarction afforded by preconditioning is mediated by A1 adenosine receptors in rabbit heart. Circulation 1991; 84: 350-356.

15.   Kuzuya T, Hoshida S, Yamashita N, et al. Delayed effects of sublethal ischemia on the acquisition of tolerance to ischemia. Circ Res 1993;72:1293-1299.

16.   Marber MS, Latchman DS, Walker JM, Yellon DM. Cardiac stress protein elevation 24 hours after brief ischemia or heat stress is associated with resistance to myocardial infarction. Circulation 1993; 88: 1264-1272.

17.   Thornton J, Striplin S, Liu GS, et al. Inhibition of protein synthesis does not block myocardial protection afforded by preconditioning. Am J Physiol 1990; 259: H1822-H1825.

18.   Hutter MM, Sievers RE, Barbosa V, Wolfe CL. Heat-shock protein induction in rat hearts. A direct correlation between the amount of heat-shock protein induced and the degree of myocardial protection. Circulation 1994; 89: 355-360.

19.   Marber MS, Walker JM, Latchman DS, Yellon DM. Myocardial protection after whole body heat stress in the rabbit is dependent on metabolic substrate and is related to the amount of inducible 70-kD heat stress protein. J Clin Invest 1994; 93: 1087-1094.

20.   Hoshida S, Kuzuya T, Fuji H, Yamashita N, et al. Sublethal ischemia alters myocardial antioxidant activity in canine heart. Am J Physiol 1993; 264: H33-H39.

21.   Nishida M, Kuzuya T, Hoshida S, Yamashita N, Hori M, Tada M. The role of manganese superoxide dismutase in the acquisition of tolerance of the heart to ischemia: molecular adaptation to ischemia. In: Maruyama Y, Hori M, Janicki JS (eds) Cardiac-Vascular Remodeling and Functional Interaction. Springer-Verlag, Tokyo. 1996; 67-77.

22.   Ambrosio G, Flaherty JT, Duilio C, et al. Oxygen radicals generated at reflow induce peroxidation of membrane lipids in reperfused hearts. J Clin Invest 1991; 87: 2056-2066.

23.   Yamashita N, Nishida M, Hoshida S, et al. Induction of manganese superoxide dismutase in rat cardiac myocytes increases tolerance to hypoxia 24 hours after preconditioning. J Clin Invest 1994; 94: 2193-2199.

24.   Currie RW, Tanguay RM, Kingma JG Jr. Heat-shock response and limitation of tissue necrosis during occlusion/reperfusion in rabbit hearts. Circulation 1993; 87: 963-971.

25.   Karmazyn M, Mailer K, Currie RW. Acquisition and decay of heat-shock-enhanced postischemic ventricular recovery. Am J Physiol 1990; 259: H424-H431.

26.   Das DK, Maulik N, Moraru II. Gene expression in acute myocardial stress. Induction by hypoxia, ischemia, reperfusion, hyperthermia and oxidative stress. J Mol Cell Cardiol 1995; 27: 181-193.

27.   Liu X, Engelman RM, Moraru II, et al. Heat shock: A new approach for myocardial preservation in cardiac surgery. Circulation 1992; 86 (suppl II): II-358-II-363.

28.   Yamashita N, Hoshida S, Nishida M, et al. Time course of tolerance to ischemia-reperfusion injury and induction of heat shock protein 72 by heat stress in the rat heart. J Mol Cell Cardiol 1997; 29: 1815-1821.

29.   Yamashita N, Hoshida S, Nishida M, et al. Heat shock-induced manganese superoxide dismutase enhances the tolerance of cardiac myocytes to hypoxia-reoxygenation injury. J Mol Cell Cardiol 1997; 29: 1805-1813.

30.   Beckmann RP, Mizzen LE, Weich WJ. Induction of HSP70 with newly synthesized protein: implications for protein folding and assembly. Science 1990; 248: 850-854.

31.   Voos W, Gambill BD, Guiard B, Pfanner N, Craig EA. Presequence and mature part of preproteins strongly influence the dependence of mitochondrial protein import on heat shock protein 70 in the matrix. J Cell Biol 1993; 123: 119-126.

32.   Suzuki K, Miura T, Sakakida S, Matsuda H. The mechanism of cardioprotective ability of heat shock protein 70; manganese superoxide dismutase is increased during ischemia-reperfusion injury in the heat shock protein 70 overexpressing heart. Circulation 1996; 94 (suppl):I-365 (abstract)

33.   Currie RW, Tanguay RM. Analysis of RNA for transcripts for catalase and SP71 in rat hearts after in vivo hyperthermia. Biochem Cell Biol. 1991; 69: 375-382.

34.   Kingma JG Jr, Simard D, Rouleau JR, Tanguay RM, Currie RW. Effect of 3-aminotriazole on hyperthermia-mediated cardioprotection in rabbits. Am J Physiol 1996; 270: H1165-H1171.

35.   Yamashita N, Nishida M, Hoshida S, et al. The protective effect of exercise on acute myocardial infarction in rat. J Am Coll Cardiol 1997; 29 (suppl): A270 (abstract).

36.   Tanaka M, Fujiwara H, Yamasaki K, Sasayama S. Superoxide dismutase and N-2-mercaptopropionyl glycine attenuate infarct size limitation effect of ischaemic preconditioning in the rabbit. Cardiovasc Res 1994; 28: 980-986.

37.   Baines CP, Goto M, Downey JM. Oxygen radicals released during ischemic preconditioning contribute to cardioprotection in the rabbit myocardium. J Mol Cell Cardiol 1997; 29: 207-216.

38.   Tritto I, D'Andrea D, Eramo N, et al. Oxygen radicals can induce preconditioning in rabbit hearts. Circ Res 1997; 80: 743-748.

39.   Chen W, Gabel S, Steenbergen C, Murphy E. A redox-based mechanism for cardioprotection induced by ischemic preconditioning in perfused rat heart. Circ Res 1995; 77: 424-429.

40.   Sun J-Z, Tang X-L, Park S-W, Qiu Y, Turrens JF, Bolli R. Evidence for an essential role of reactive oxygen species in the genesis of late preconditioning against myocardial stunning in conscious pigs. J Clin Invest 1996; 97: 562-576.

41.   Yamashita N, Hoshida S, Taniguchi N, Kuzuya T, Hori M. A "second window of protection" occurs 24 hours after ischemic preconditioning in rat heart. J Mol Cell Cardiol 1998; in press.

42.   Oberley LW, St.Clair DK, Autor AP, Oberley TD. Increase in manganese superoxide dismutase activity in the mouse heart after x-irradiation. Arch Biochem Biophys 1987; 254: 69-80.

43.   Warner BB, Stuart L, Gebb S, Wispe JR. Redox regulation of manganese superoxide dismutase. Am J Physiol 1996; 271: L150-L158.

44.   Zhou X, Zhai X, Ashraf M. Direct evidence that initial oxidtaive stress triggered by preconditioning contributes to second window of protection by endogenous antioxidant enzyme in myocytes. Circulation 1996; 93: 1177-1184.

9

Endotoxin, Monophosphoryl Lipid A and Delayed Cardioprotection

G J Gross

1. Introduction

In 1989, Brown and colleagues [1] demonstrated that pretreatment of rats with a low dose of endotoxin (lipopolysaccharide, LPS) 24 hours prior to heart isolation and perfusion in the Langendorff mode resulted in an enhanced post-ischaemic recovery of myocardial function (left ventricular developed pressure, + dP/dt) and an increase in catalase activity. Hearts isolated from rats which were pretreated with LPS for only 1 hour did not have an increased catalase activity or functional protection from ischaemia-reperfusion injury. These results suggested that the delayed cardioprotection produced by LPS was the result of enhanced antioxidant enzyme activity, particularly catalase.

More recently, Rowland and co-workers [2] and Meng et al. [3] showed that LPS administered at 500 µg/kg, intraperitoneally, to rats 72 hours prior to heart isolation and subjecting it to 20 minutes of global ischaemia and reperfusion for 30 minutes resulted in an enhanced recovery of function and a reduction in creatine kinase (CK) release during reperfusion. These results suggested that LPS produced a delayed cardioprotective effect to reduce stunning (enhanced function) and to decrease cellular necrosis (CK release). The magnitude of cardioprotection was similar to that observed following a 5 minute period of ischaemic preconditioning (PC). Furthermore, these investigators found that when LPS pretreated hearts were concomitantly subjected to acute PC the effects were greater than those observed when either stimulus was used alone which suggested that these stimuli may be producing cardioprotection by separate mechanisms (Figure 1). However, in spite of these interesting results obtained with LPS, this

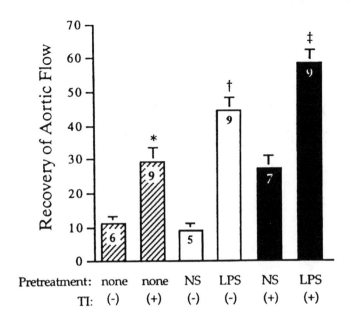

Figure 1. Percent recovery of aortic low after ischaemia and reperfusion in isolated rat hearts. Recovery based on end reperfusion (30 min) aortic flow relative to baseline pre-ischaemic values. Recoveries for TI (transient ischaemia = preconditioning) and LPS + TI are based on aortic flows in the equilibration period before the 5-min ischaemic interval. Acute preconditioning involved no pretreatment. Pretreatment for delayed protection experiments involved normal saline (NS, controls) or LPS administration 72h before heart isolation. Percent recoveries for each treated group were significantly greater than for their respective controls. LPS-induced recovery of aortic flow was greater than the recovery seen with TI alone. Combining LPS with TI (acute + delayed) resulted in the greatest aortic flow recovery relative to TI or LPS separately. Values are means ± SE. *P<0.05 vs. ischaemic control; †P<0.05 vs. LPS control (NS alone), TI; ‡P<0.05 vs LPS + TI control (saline + TI), LPS. Numbers in bars represent n per group. Reproduced by permission of the American Physiological Society and by the American Journal of Physiology 1997; 272: H2708-H2715.

compound is known to produce toxic side effects, such as neutrophil activation, diffuse intravascular coagulation and pyrogenicity which would limit its use in a clinical setting. Therefore, there have been numerous attempts at modifying the LPS molecule in an attempt to synthesise an analogue which would retain the cardioprotective properties of LPS without its associated toxic potential. In this regard, Qureshi et al. [4] synthesised and purified an endotoxin derivative named monophosphoryl lipid A (MLA, Figure 2) and Ribi [5] found that MLA is considerably less toxic than LPS. More recently, MLA has been shown to possess marked cardioprotective activity in a number of animal models [6-9] and this chapter will attempt to summarise the results of these studies and several recent ones with LPS [2,3] and address potential mechanisms that may be responsible for the beneficial effects of MLA and LPS.

2. Effects of MLA and LPS on Myocardial Infarct Size

Initial studies performed by Yao et al. [6,7] in pentobarbitone-anaesthetised dogs, demonstrated that 24 hour pretreatment with MLA (30-100µg/kg, iv) produced a significant reduction in myocardial infarct size. However, no reduction in infarct size was observed after one hour pretreatment which suggested that a finite period of time longer than 60 minutes was necessary for the cardioprotective effect of MLA to be manifest. These results are similar to those obtained by Brown et al. [1] using LPS in rats in which they also found to be effective at enhancing functional recovery following 24 hours but not 1 hour of pretreatment. Similarly, reductions in infarct size following 24 hours of pretreatment with MLA have been observed by Elliott et al. [8], Przyklenk et al. [9], Baxter et al. [10] and Yoshida et al. [11] in anaesthetized dogs and rabbits. Interestingly, Baxter et al. [10] did not observe a reduction in infarct size in isolated buffer-perfused rabbit hearts 24 hours after MLA pretreatment. These authors concluded that the protection afforded by MLA was only observed in vivo possibly because its delayed effect may be mediated by humoral or blood-borne factors (see below).

Although the cardioprotective effects of MLA were not observed following one hour of pretreatment, recent preliminary results of Weber et al. [12] demonstrated that MLA produced an acute or early phase of cardioprotection in anaesthetized rabbits which persisted for only 10-20 minutes and returned 12-24 hours later. These results are similar to those obtained with ischaemic PC in which there is also a short-lived cardioprotective effect subsequent to single or multiple brief periods of ischaemia and reperfusion (known as early, acute or classic PC) followed by a second window of protection (called SWOP, or delayed PC) 12-24 hours later [13,14]. However, whereas SWOP produced by brief periods of ischaemia generally produces a reduction in infarct size of approximately 50%, classic ischaemic PC usually results in a 75-80% reduction. In this regard, Mei et al. [15] recently found that MLA-induced SWOP resulted in a reduction in infarct size similar to that of classic ischaemic PC (75%) which suggests that delayed protection produced by MLA has a greater cardioprotective effect than SWOP induced by ischaemia; it may, therefore, may be of greater potential clinical benefit. A recent study of Eising et al. [16] in intact rats demonstrated that repeated exposure to low doses of LPS for 7 days prior to a 45 minute coronary artery occlusion and 3 days of reperfusion

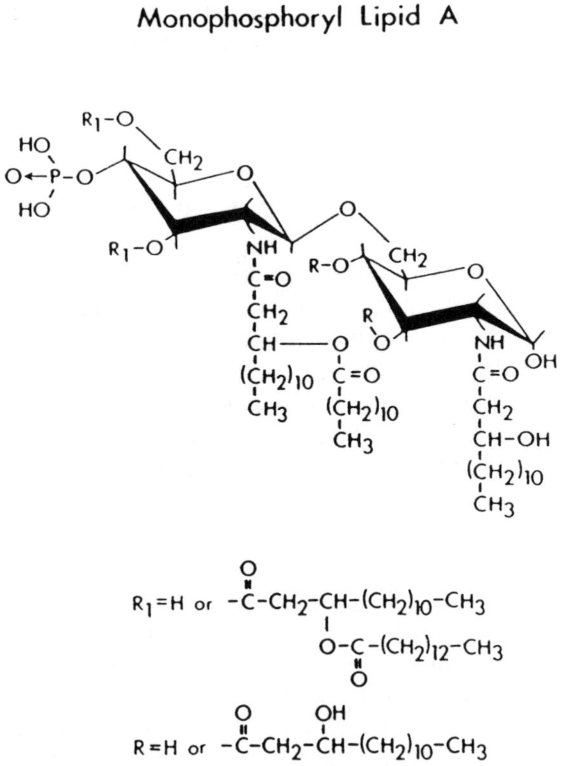

Monophosphoryl Lipid A

Figure 2. Chemical structure of monophosphoryl lipid A (MLA)

also resulted in a significant reduction in infarct size (Figure 3). The magnitude of this effect (37% decrease) was considerably less than that normally observed with MLA (50-75% decrease) in infarct models. However, no direct comparisons have been made between MLA and LPS in a rat model. Nevertheless, these data suggest that both low dose LPS and MLA have a delayed cardioprotective effect in several animal models of myocardial infarction.

3. Effects of MLA and LPS on Myocardial Stunning

Single or multiple brief periods (5-20 minutes) of myocardial ischaemia followed by reperfusion have been shown to result in prolonged, reversible abnormalities in regional systolic or diastolic contractile function, a phenomenon known as stunned myocardium [17]. Evidence to suggest that MLA might effectively attenuate post-ischaemic contractile dysfunction was first obtained by Nelson et al. [18]. These

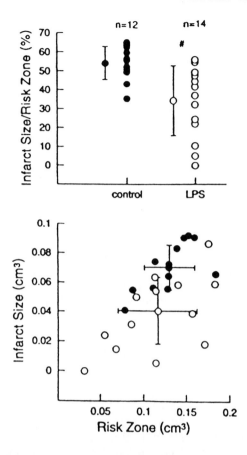

Figure 3. Upper panel is a scatter plot of infarct size expressed as a percent of the area at risk for control rats (control) and for lipopolysaccharide-tolerant rats (LPS). There was a significant (#P<0.002) decrease in infarct size in the LPS tolerant group. Lower panel depicts the risk zone plotted versus infarct size in control (solid circles) and LPS-tolerant animals (open circles). Although there is some overlap, the control infarct size points are generally higher regardless of risk zone size. Reproduced by permission of Elsevier Science B.V., The Netherlands and Cardiovascular Research 1996; 31: 73-81.

investigators found that 24 hours of pretreatment with MLA resulted in enhanced recovery of developed pressure in isolated buffer-perfused rat hearts subjected to global ischaemia and reperfusion. In agreement, Zhao, et al. [19] also found that 24 hour pretreatment with MLA resulted in a significant improvement in left ventricular developed pressure, dP/dt, rate-pressure product and mean arterial pressure following 90 minutes of regional ischaemia and 6 hours of reperfusion in anaesthetised rabbits.

Yao et al. [20] were the first to determine the effect of MLA in a classic model of regional myocardial stunning in anaesthetised dogs. Systolic segment shortening (%SS) was determined by ultrasonic dimension gauges implanted in the subendocardium of three groups of animals, controls and those pretreated with MLA 1 or 24 hours prior to stunning. Regional segment dysfunction was produced by six 5 minute periods of coronary artery occlusion interspersed with 10 minute periods of reperfusion and finally by 2 hours of reperfusion. Pretreatment with MLA one hour prior to the first occlusion period had no effect on the recovery of %SS. However, pretreatment for 24 hours resulted in an enhanced recovery of %SS during all reperfusion periods as compared to the control group (Figure 4). Thus, 24 hour pretreatment with MLA has been shown to be cardioprotective in models of both irreversible and reversible myocardial injury in various animal species. Similarly, 24-72 hours of pretreatment with low dose of LPS has also been shown to attenuate stunning in isolated rat hearts [1-3]. Potential mechanisms by which these protective effects occur will be addressed next and include a possible role for neutrophils, heat shock proteins, K_{ATP} channels, adenosine and nitric oxide (NO).

4. Role of Neutrophils In MLA- and LPS-induced Infarct Size Reduction

Although a role for neutrophil activation in the pathogenesis of stunned myocardium has been clearly shown to not exist [21], numerous studies suggest that polymorphonuclear leukocytes may be important in determining ultimate infarct size in models of prolonged ischaemia followed by reperfusion [22]. Yao et al. [6] showed that MLA pretreatment for 24 hours resulted in a marked decrease in myeloperoxidase (MPO) activity, an index of neutrophil infiltration, in the border zone surrounding infarcted tissue in canine hearts (Figure 5). More recently, Zhao et al. [23] found a similar effect of MLA to decrease MPO activity in the border zone surrounding the infarct area in anaesthetised rabbits. Similarly, Eising et al. [16] found 3 days after coronary artery occlusion and reperfusion that the percent of activated neutrophils was markedly reduced in LPS-pretreated rats (2.9 ± 1.6 vs. 11.4 ± 7.2%, respectively).

It is unknown if the reduction in MPO activity and neutrophil activation observed in LPS- and MLA-treated animals is a primary event related to an action of LPS or MLA on neutrophil or endothelial cell adhesion molecules or a secondary event related to the smaller infarct size. The cardioprotective effect of MLA to reduce infarct size in rabbits and decrease MPO activity, were both blocked by a selective inhibitor of inducible nitric oxide synthase (NOS), aminoguanidine [23], which

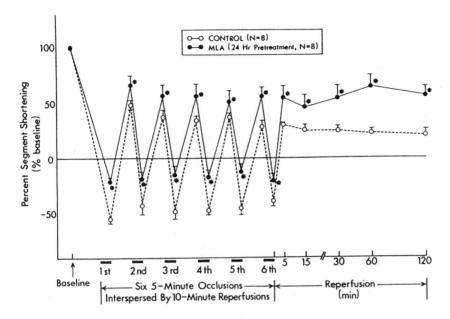

Figure 4. Pretreatment with monophosphoryl lipid A (MLA, 35μg/kg, iv) 24 hours prior to six 5 minute coronary artery occlusions followed by 2 hours of reperfusion markedly improved the recovery of regional systolic shortening (%SS) throughout all occlusion and reperfusion periods. *P<0.05 versus the control group. All values are the mean ± SEM (N = 8, each group). Reproduced with permission of S. Karger AG, Basel, Switzerland and Pharmacology 1995; 51: 152-159.

suggests that MLA may be enhancing nitric oxide (NO) production. In this regard, it is well-known that NO has beneficial effects to block neutrophil activation and infiltration into ischaemic-reperfused myocardium [24].

5. Role of Heat Shock Proteins in MLA- and LPS-induced Cardioprotection

Recent studies have suggested that heat shock proteins (HSPs) may be involved in the delayed cardioprotection observed in hearts subjected to various stresses such as ischaemia, high temperature and oxygen-derived free radicals [25]. These proteins are highly conserved and there is evidence that LPS results in increased synthesis of HSP70 in rat hearts

[26]. Based upon these results with LPS, two laboratories [10, 11] investigated the effect of 24 hour pretreatment with MLA on the expression of HSP 70 in rabbit hearts. In both studies, MLA pretreatment resulted in a marked reduction in myocardial infarct size in anaesthetised rabbits subjected to 30 minutes of regional ischaemia followed by 24 hours of reperfusion. However, there was no evidence for an increased expression of the inducible form of HSP70 by Western blot analysis. However, heat stress did enhance the expression of HSP 70 in both studies. These results suggest that MLA does not appear to produce its cardioprotective effects via increased concentrations of HSPs although it is still possible that an increase in small molecular weight HSPs might occur. More likely, MLA is acting via a novel signalling pathway that does not involve HSPs. Studies specifically addressing the role of HSPs in the cardioprotective actions of LPS have not been performed, although it is known that LPS treatment results in increased expression of HSPs [10, 16, 26].

6. Role of ATP-Sensitive Potassium Channels (K_{ATP}) In MLA-induced Infarct Size Reduction

In 1992, Gross and Auchampach [27] were the first to describe an important role for the K_{ATP} channel in mediating the cardioprotective effect of classic ischaemic PC in the canine heart. They found that the marked infarct size reducing effect of PC was completely abolished by administration of the K_{ATP} channel blocker glibenclamide either before or after PC which suggested that K_{ATP} channel activation was responsible for both triggering as well as maintaining the preconditioned state. The K_{ATP} channel opener aprikalim also mimicked the cardioprotective effect of PC [27]. Since MLA produced a reduction in infarct size similar in magnitude to that of classic PC, it was hypothesized that the K_{ATP} channel might also be an important component of its cardioprotective effect. Therefore, we examined the effect of MLA to reduce infarct size in dogs and further examined the role of the K_{ATP} channel in mediating the beneficial effect of MLA by pretreating animals with either glibenclamide or 5-hydroxydecanoic acid (5-HD), two structurally dissimilar K_{ATP} channel blockers [15]. MLA administered at either 3, 10 or 35 µg/kg 24 hours prior to a 60 minute occlusion period resulted in a marked and dose-related reduction in myocardial infarct size with a significant reduction observed at 10 and 35 µg/kg (Figure 6). Furthermore, the cardioprotective effect of MLA was completely abolished by pretreatment with glibenclamide or 5-HD. Similarly, Elliott and coworkers [8] recently found nearly identical results in an anaesthetised rabbit infarct model. They found that 10 and 35 µg/kg of MLA produced nearly equivalent reductions in infarct size of 64 and 71% and that the effect of the high dose (35 µg/kg) was

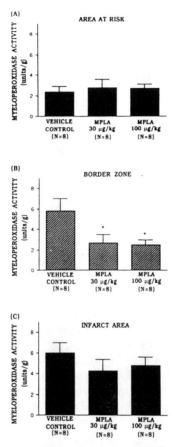

Figure 5. Effects of monophosphoryl lipid A (MPLA) on myeloperoxidase (MPO) activity in the area at risk distant from the infarct, the border zone surrounding the infarct and the central ischaemic zone in canine myocardium. There was a significant reduction in MPO activity in the border zone in the group pretreated with MLA (30 and 100 µg/kg, iv) 24 hours prior to the prolonged ischaemic period. *P<0.05 versus the control group. Reproduced by permission of Elsevier Sciences B.V., The Netherlands and Cardiovascular Research 1993; 27: 832-838.

completely blocked by pretreatment with glibenclamide (0.3 mg/kg, iv). These results were the first to implicate a role for the K_{ATP} channel in delayed protection and suggest that the K_{ATP} channel may be the end effector of both early and delayed PC. In this regard, preliminary results from Kukreja's laboratory [28] have shown that delayed PC produced in rabbit hearts by four 5 minute occlusions performed 24 hours prior to a prolonged ischaemic period was blocked by glibenclamide and 5-HD which suggests that both early and delayed PC are mediated by the opening of K_{ATP} channels, at least in rabbit hearts.

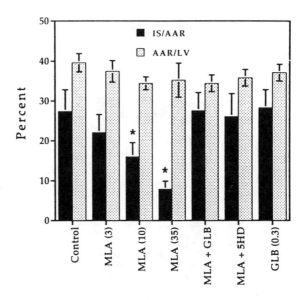

Figure 6. Infarct size expressed as a percent of the area at risk (IS/AAR) and area at risk expressed as a percent of left ventricular weight (AAR/LV). All doses of MLA are expressed in µg/kg. Values are the mean ± SEM (N = 7-8 dogs/group). MLA produced a dose-dependent decrease in IS/AAR that was blocked by the K_{ATP} antagonists glibenclamide (0.3mg/kg, iv) or 5-hydroxydecanoic acid (5-HD, 7.5 mg/kg, ic). *P<0.05 as compared to the control group. Reproduced by permission of the American Physiological Society and by the American Journal of Physiology 1996; 271: H2723-H2729.

7. Role of K_{ATP} Channels In MLA-induced Attenuation Of Stunning

Since the K_{ATP} channel has been shown to be a key mediator in the cardioprotective effect of MLA to reduce infarct size in dogs, we hypothesised that enhanced activation of the K_{ATP} channel might also be important in mediating its anti-stunning effect. Therefore, a study was designed to determine the effect of MLA to enhance regional systolic shortening (%SS) in stunned myocardium and to determine the role of the K_{ATP} channel in mediating the cardioprotective effect of MLA in anaesthetized dogs. To produce myocardial stunning, dogs were subjected to 5 periods of 5 minutes of left anterior descending coronary artery occlusion interspersed with 10 minutes of reperfusion and finally followed by 2 hours of reperfusion. MLA in a range of 10-35 µg/kg given 24 hours prior to ischaemia resulted in an improvement in %SS with a maximal protective effect obtained at 10 µg/kg. The cardioprotective effect of MLA (10 µg/kg) was completely blocked by the K_{ATP} channel blocker glibenclamide (Figure 7) at a dose (50 µg/kg) which had no effect on stunning in control animals. These results suggest that MLA improves %SS by a KATP channel-dependent mechanism and that MLA mimics the anti-stunning effects observed during ischaemia-induced delayed preconditioning. Since adenosine and NO have been implicated as endogenous mediators in delayed PC [23, 29] and have also been shown to enhance the activation of K_{ATP} channels [30,31] the role that these two mediators play in the cardioprotective effect of MLA will be discussed next.

8. Role of Adenosine In the Cardioprotective Effect of MLA

The first study to suggest that adenosine might be involved in the cardioprotective effect of MLA was provided by Zhao et al. [19]. These investigators found that 24 hour pretreatment with MLA improved the recovery of contractile function in rabbit hearts exposed to 90 minutes of regional ischaemia and reperfusion and that this improvement in function was associated with a preservation of ATP and ADP and an increase in adenosine kinase activity in normal and post-ischaemic myocardium. It was hypothesised that the increase in adenosine kinase activity might result in an increased recycling of adenosine to AMP, ADP and ATP and these effects might be responsible for the improvement in functional recovery in MLA-pretreated hearts.

Another enzyme which has been proposed to be important in the development of early PC against infarction is 5'-nucleotidase (5'-NT), the enzyme that catalyses the formation of adenosine from 5'-AMP [9]. Kitakaze et al. [32] have shown that blockade of 5'-NT by α, β-methylene adenosine 5'-diphosphate (AOPCP) attenuated the infarct limiting effect of early PC produced by ischaemia. Since there is some evidence to suggest that MLA increases 5'-NT activity in humans [33], it was hypothesized that MLA might produce its cardioprotective effect via this mechanism. In this regard, Przyklenk et al. [9] tested the effect of both ischaemia-induced classic PC and MLA-induced delayed protection to reduce infarct size and attempted to correlate the magnitude of the reduction in infarct size produced by these two interventions to increases in 5'-NT activity in anaesthetized dogs. Interestingly, both ischaemic PC and MLA pretreatment resulted in increases in 5'-NT activity. However, single and multivariate regression analyses found that there was no significant correlation between infarct size reduction and increases in 5'-NT activity. Surprisingly, the hearts with the largest infarcts had the greatest 5'-NT activity. Therefore, these authors concluded that increases in 5'-NT activity were not primarily responsible for the cardioprotective effect of MLA or ischaemic PC in

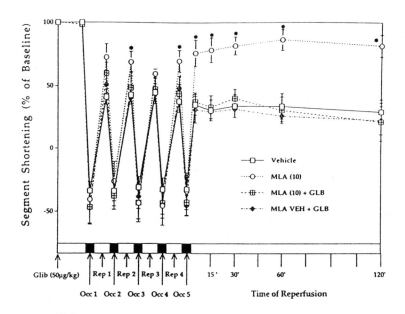

Figure 7. Pretreatment with the K_{ATP} antagonist, glibenclamide (50 μg/kg, iv) 15 minutes prior to myocardial stunning completely blocked the cardioprotective effect of MLA (10 μg/kg, iv) given 24 hours prior to ischaemia. This dose of glibenclamide had no effect in vehicle-treated controls. All values are the mean ± SEM (N = 6-8/group). *P<0.05 MLA (10) versus vehicle-treated controls.

canine hearts. Although adenosine concentrations were not measured, these results also suggested that increases in adenosine were not responsible for the infarct size-reducing effect of these two interventions.

Preliminary results recently obtained by Mei et al. [34] in dogs compared the effect of early ischaemic PC to that of delayed PC produced by MLA on infarct size and interstitial levels of adenosine and its purine breakdown products prior to ischaemia, during ischaemic PC, during a 60 minute occlusion period and throughout the first 30 minutes of reperfusion. In both MLA-pretreated and ischaemic preconditioned animals there was a significant reduction in myocardial infarct size and interstitial adenosine was elevated prior to the prolonged ischaemic period. However, there was a marked decrease in interstitial adenosine during the 60 minute ischaemic period and during the first 30 minutes of reperfusion in both treated groups. Since we have recently shown that adenosine is only a trigger for ischaemic PC in dogs [35], it is likely that the increases in adenosine observed prior to the prolonged ischaemic period in both MLA and ischaemic preconditioned dogs are sufficient to sensitise the K_{ATP} channel to open more readily or to a greater extent during the 60 minute occlusion period. That ischaemic PC and MLA both produce a similar reduction in infarct size and interstitial purines during the prolonged ischaemic period suggests but does not prove a common mechanism of action for these two interventions. Further studies with selective adenosine receptor antagonists are needed in MLA-pretreated animals to define more clearly a key role for adenosine in its cardioprotective effect.

9. Role of NO in MLA-induced Cardioprotection

LPS has been previously shown to induce the synthesis of inducible NOS [26]. Similarly, Gustafson and Rhodes [31] have also demonstrated that MLA induces NOS in some cells and it is possible that MLA enhances NO production in endothelial cells and/or the myocardium thereby resulting in a reduction in neutrophil infiltration into the reperfused region which would lead to a decrease in reperfusion injury and ultimate infarct size. Zhao and coworkers [23] recently directly tested the hypothesis that MLA pretreatment mimics SWOP in anaesthetised rabbit hearts by upregulating inducible NOS. MLA pretreatment significantly reduced myocardial infarct size and reduced neutrophil infiltration into the border zone surrounding the infarcted area. Aminoguanidine (300 mg/kg, SC), a selective inducible NOS inhibitor, given one hour prior to a 30 minute occlusion period completely blocked the infarct size limiting effect of MLA and attenuated the reduction in neutrophil infiltration. MLA also produced a small increase in inducible NOS enzyme activity in the post-ischaemic area as compared to the non-ischaemic area at 15 and 30 minutes after the induction of ischaemia. Since Cameron and coworkers [37] and Shinbo and Iijima [31] have both shown that NO enhances K_{ATP} channel activity using patch clamp techniques in cardiac myocytes, these findings suggest that a link may exist between enhanced NO production and increased K_{ATP} channel activity in MLA-pretreated animals and provides a unifying mechanism by which this agent produces a cardioprotective effect against infarction and stunning. Whether similar mechanisms are involved in mediating the cardioprotective effects of low dose LPS are not known and require further investigation.

10. Conclusion

MLA and LPS pretreatment 24-72 hours prior to a brief or prolonged ischaemic insult have been shown to produce a cardioprotective effect against both myocardial infarction and stunning. The mechanism responsible for the cardioprotective effect of MLA appears to be mediated via enhanced activation of the K_{ATP} channel. Increased induction of NOS appears to be an important component of the signalling pathway leading to increased K_{ATP} channel activity, whereas a role for adenosine is less apparent. Other signalling pathways such as protein kinase C or tyrosine kinases have yet to be thoroughly investigated but future research will undoubtedly uncover more pieces of the puzzle which are involved in mediating the cardioprotective effects of LPS and MLA. The results obtained thus far in animals and in preliminary clinical trials in man suggest that compounds such as MLA may have a number of therapeutic applications in cardiovascular medicine.

Acknowledgements

This work was supported by NIH Grant HL 08311 and a contract from RIBI ImmunoChem, Inc., Hamilton, Montana, USA. The authors wishes to thank Donna Sloane for excellent secretarial assistance and Jeannine Moore and Anna Hsu for excellent technical assistance.

References

1.   Brown JM., Gross MA, Terada LS et al. Endotoxin pretreatment increases endogenous myocardial catalase activity and decreases ischemia-reperfusion injury of isolated rat hearts. Proc Nat Acad Sci USA 86: 2516-2520. 1989.

2.   Rowland RT, Meng X, Cleveland JC Jr, Meldrum DR, Harken AH, Brown JM LPS-induced delayed myocardial adaptation enhances acute preconditioning to optimize postischemic cardiac function. Am J Physiol. 272: H2708-H2715, 1997.

3.   Meng X, Ao L Brown JM et al. LPS induces late cardiac functional protection against ischemia independent of cardiac and circulating TNF-α. Am J Physiol. 273: H1894-H1902, 1997.

4.   Qureshi N, TakayamaK, Ribi,E. Purification and structural determination of nontoxic lipid A obtained from lipopolysaccharide of salmonella typhimurium. J Biol Chem.257: 11808-11815, 1982.

5.   Ribi E. Beneficial modification of the endotoxin molecule. J.Biol Resp Modif 3: 1-9, 1984.

6.   Yao Z, Auchampach JA, Pieper GM, Gross GJ. Cardioprotective effect of monophosphoryl lipid A, a novel endotoxin analogue, in dogs. Cardiovasc Res 27: 832-838, 1993.

7.   Yao Z, Rasmussen JR, Hirt JL, Mei DA, Pieper GM, Gross GJ. Effects of monophosphoryl lipid A on myocardial ischemia/reperfusion injury and vascular endothelial and smooth muscle function in dogs. J Cardiovasc Pharmacol 22: 653-663, 1993.

8.   Elliott GT, Comerford ML, Smith JR, Zhao, L. Myocardial ischemia/reperfusion protection using monophosphoryl lipid A is abrogated by the ATP-sensitive potassium channel blocker, glibenclamide. Cardiovasc Res 32: 1071-1080, 1996.

9.   Przyklenk K, Zhao L, Kloner RA, Elliott GT. Cardioprotection with ischemic preconditioning and MLA: role of adenosine-regulating enzymes? Am J Physiol 271: H1004-H1014, 1996.

10.   Baxter GF, Goodwin RW, Wright MJ, Kerac M, Heads RJ, Yellon DM. Myocardial protection after monophosphoryl lipid A: studies of delayed anti-ischaemic properties in rabbit hearts. Br J Pharmacol 117: 1685-1692, 1996.

11.   Yoshida K, Maajeh MM, Shipley JB et al. Monophosphoryl lipid A induces pharmacologic preconditioning in rabbit hearts without concomitant expression of 70-kDa heat shock protein. Mol Cell Biochem 159: 73-80, 1996.

12.   Weber P, Smart M, Comerford M, Smith J, Zhao L, Elliott G. Monophosphoryl lipid A mimics both first and second window of ischemic preconditioning and preserves myocardial sarcoplasmic reticular calcium pump. J. Mol. Cell. Cardiol. 29: A233, 1997 (abstract).

13.   Yellon DM, Baxter GF. A "second window of protection" or delayed preconditioning phenomenon: future horizons for myocardial protection. J Mol Cell Cardiol 27: 1023-1034, 1995.

14.   BaxterGF, Goma FM, Yellon DM. Characterization of the infarct-limiting effect of delayed preconditioning: time course and dose-dependency studies in rabbit myocardium. Basic Res Cardiol 92: 159-167, 1997.

15.   Mei DA, Elliott GT, Gross GJ. K_{ATP} channels mediate late preconditioning against infarction produced by monophosphoryl lipid A. Am J Physiol 271: H2723-H2729, 1996.

16.   Eising GP, Mao L, Schmid-Schonbein GW, Engler RL, Ross J. Effects of induced tolerance to bacterial lipopolysaccharide on myocardial infarct size in rats. Cardiovasc Res 31: 73-81. 1996.

17.   Braunwald E, Kloner RA. The stunned myocardium: prolonged postischemic ventricular dysfunction. Circulation 66: 1146-1149, 1982.

18.   Nelson DW, Brown JM, Banerjee A et al. Pretreatment with a nontoxic derivative of endotoxin induces functional protection against cardiac ischemia/reperfusion injury. Surgery 110: 365-369, 1991.

19.   Zhao L, Kirsch CC, Hagen SR, Elliott GT. Preservation of global cardiac function in the rabbit following protracted ischemia/reperfusion using monophosphoryl lipid A (MLA). J Mol. Cell Cardiol 28: 197-208, 1996.

20.   Yao Z, Elliot GT, Gross GJ. Monophosphoryl lipid A preserves myocardial contractile function following multiple, brief periods of coronary occlusion in dogs. Pharmacology 51: 152-159, 1995.

21.   Jeremy RW, Becker LC. Neutrophil depletion does not prevent myocardial dysfunction after brief coronary occlusion. J Am Coll Cardiol 13: 1155-1163, 1989.

22.   Hansen PR. Role of neutrophils in myocardial ischemia and reperfusion. Circulation 91: 1872-1885, 1995.

23.   Zhao L, Weber PA, Smith JR, Comerford ML, Elliott GT. Role of inducible nitric oxide synthase in pharmacological "preconditioning" with monophosphoryl lipid A. J Mol Cell Cardiol 29: 1567-1576, 1997.

24.   Pieper GM, Clarke GA, Gross GJ. Stimulatory and inhibitory action of nitric oxide donor agents vs. nitrovasodilators on reactive oxygen production by isolated polymorphonuclear leukocytes. J Pharmacol Exp Ther 269: 451-456, 1994.

25.   Marber MS, Mestril R, Chi SH, Sayen MR, Yellon DM, Dillmann WH. A heat shock protein 70 transgene results in myocardial protection. J Clin Invest 95: 1446-1456, 1995.

26.   Zingarelli B, Halushka PV, Caputi AP, Cook JA. Increased nitric oxide synthase during the development of endotoxin tolerance. Shock 3: 102-108,1995.

27.   Gross GJ, Auchampach JA. Blockade of ATP-sensitive potassium channels prevents myocardial preconditioning in dogs. Circ.Res 1992; 70: 223-233, 1992.

28.   Bernardo NL, D'Angelo M, Desai PV, Levasseur JE, Kukreja RC. ATP-sensitive potassium channel is involved in the second window of ischemic preconditioning in rabbit. J Mol Cell Cardiol 29: 293, 1997.

29.   Baxter GF, Marber MS, Patel VC, Yellon DM. Adenosine receptor involvement in a delayed phase of myocardial protection 24 hours after ischemic preconditioning. Circulation 90: 2993-3000, 1994.

30.   Kim E, Han J, Ho W, Earm YE. Modulation of ATP-sensitive K+ channels in rabbit ventricular myocytes by adenosine A1 receptor activation. Am J Physiol 272: H325-H333, 1997.

31.   Shinbo A, Iijima T. Potentiation by nitric oxide of the ATP-sensitive K+ current induced by K+ channel openers in guinea pig ventricular cells. Br J Pharmacol 120: 1568-1574, 1997.

32.　　Kitakaze M, Hori M, Morioka T et al. Infarct size-limiting effect of ischemic preconditioning is blunted by inhibition of 5'-nucleotidase activity and attenuation of adenosine release. Circulation 89: 1237-1246, 1994.

33.　　Astiz ME, Rackow EC, Still JG. Pretreatment of normal humans with monophosphoryl lipid A induces tolerance to endotoxin: a prospective, double-blind, randomized, controlled trial. Crit Care Med 23: 9-17, 1995.

34.　　Mei DA, Elliott GT, Gross GJ. Comparative effects of early ischemic preconditioning (PC) and late PC induced by monophosphoryl lipid A upon myocardial infarct size and interstitial purine metabolism in dogs. Circulation 94: 1072, 1996 (abstract).

35.　　Yao Z, Mizumura T, Mei DA, Gross GJ. K_{ATP} channels and memory of ischemic preconditioning in dogs: synergism between adenosine and KATP channels. Am J Physiol 272: H334-H342, 1997.

36.　　Gustafson GL, Rhodes MJ. A rationale for the prophylactic use of monophosphoryl lipid A in sepsis and septic shock. Biochem Biophys Res Commun 182: 269-275, 1992.

37.　　Cameron JS, Kibler KKA, Berry H, Barron DN, Sodder VH. Nitric oxide activates ATP-sensitive potassium channels in hypertrophied ventricular myocytes. FASEB J 10: A65, 1996 (abstract).

10

Adenosine and Delayed Cardioprotection

A Dana, D M Yellon and G F Baxter

1. Introduction

Adenosine is a purine nucleoside that is produced by catabolism of adenosine triphosphate (ATP) by many different cell types. The cardiovascular actions of adenosine have been appreciated for many years (see reference 1 for review). It is known that various forms of myocardial stress, including ischaemia, hypoxia or catecholamines, result in a rapid increase in extracellular levels of adenosine. This in turn results in activation of local adenosine receptors on cardiomyocytes and vascular endothelial cells which mediate a reduction in metabolic demand of the heart and an increase in myocardial oxygen supply by coronary vasodilatation. These observations have led to the concept that adenosine is a "retaliatory metabolite" with potential cardioprotective effects [2]. Due to the efficient transport mechanisms and metabolising enzymes, the effects of adenosine are localised to the site where it is formed; the duration of its effects are very transient with a half-life in human blood of less than one second [3]. Thus adenosine is considered a short-term mediator that maintains the metabolic equilibrium of the heart within a time frame of seconds to minutes.

In the past few years it has been recognised that in addition to these short-term effects, adenosine may provoke cellular adaptive responses that may manifest over a period of several hours. For example it has been shown that adenosine released during a brief period of sublethal ischaemia acts as both the trigger, provoking the cellular events that lead to protection, and the mediator of classic ischaemic preconditioning [4]. More recent work has indicated that signalling via adenosine receptors can also regulate the expression of a number of genes, thereby prolonging the consequences of adenosine receptor activation beyond the short half-life of adenosine itself. Adenosine has been reported to mediate both increases (for example vascular endothelial growth factor) [5] and decreases (for example tumour necrosis factor) [6] in gene expression. In view of these findings, and the fact that brief preconditioning ischaemia is a powerful stimulus for increasing extracellular levels of adenosine, we hypothesised that as with classic preconditioning, adenosine may be an important trigger for the delayed phase of myocardial protection which is observed many hours after the preconditioning stimulus. In this chapter we summarise the evidence for the role of adenosine in triggering this 'second window of protection' and the current knowledge regarding potential signalling mechanisms downstream of adenosine receptors.

2. Adenosine as a Trigger of Delayed Preconditioning

Initially, we examined a potential role for adenosine in triggering the delayed phase of cardioprotection following ischaemic preconditioning [7]. Rabbits were anaesthetised and subjected to a preconditioning protocol of four 5 minute coronary artery occlusions and 10 minute reperfusion. During this protocol animals were also treated with an intravenous infusion of 8-(p-sulphophenyl)-theophylline (SPT), a non-selective adenosine receptor antagonist, or saline. Twenty four hours after this pretreatment, animals were subjected to an infarction protocol consisting of 30 minutes coronary artery occlusion and 2 hours reperfusion after which infarct size was assessed with triphenyltetrazolium chloride (TTC) staining. Similar to our previous results [8], ischaemic preconditioning resulted in a significant and sustained limitation of infarct size compared to sham operated controls (figure 1). Furthermore, we found that inhibition of adenosine receptors during the preconditioning protocol with SPT completely abolished the cardioprotective effects observed at 24 hours, implying a role for adenosine receptors in triggering delayed protection against myocardial infarction. In the same group of experiments we substituted the preconditioning protocol with either a single intravenous bolus of the highly selective adenosine A_1 receptor agonist 2-chloro-N^6-cyclopentyladenosine (CCPA) or saline vehicle. Increasing doses of CCPA in the range 25 to 100 µg/kg resulted in progressive reduction of infarct size compared to saline treated animals with the maximum protection observed with the 100 µg/kg dose producing a 50% reduction in infarct/risk ratio (figure 2). These results clearly implicate a role for adenosine A_1 receptors in triggering the delayed infarct limiting effects of ischaemic preconditioning in the rabbit.

Since these original experiments, we have confirmed our findings in our in vivo infarct model [9, 10], and also in isolated Langendorff

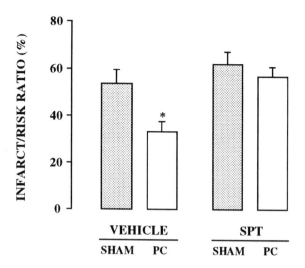

Figure 1. Effects of adenosine receptor blockade on delayed preconditioning in the rabbit. Rabbits were preconditioned (PC) or sham operated (SHAM). During this period, they received either 8-(p-sulphophenyl)-theophylline (SPT) or vehicle (saline). After 24 hours they were subjected to 30 minutes coronary artery occlusion and infarct size was determined by TTC staining. SPT completely abolished the delayed protective effects of preconditioning, suggesting that endogenous adenosine is a trigger of adaptation. * P < 0.05 vs vehicle SHAM. Adapted from Circulation 1994; 90: 2993-3000 with permission.

perfused rabbit hearts [11] thereby excluding a contribution by systemic neurohormonal or blood-borne elements to the delayed cardioprotective effects of adenosine A_1 rteceptor activation. Recent preliminary data from our laboratory indicate that A_1 receptor agonists induce a similar delayed protection against infarction in the rat heart. Animals treated with a single intravenous bolus of CCPA 100 µg/kg had significantly smaller infarct sizes (expressed as a percentage of area at risk) compared to saline treated controls when subjected to 35 minutes regional myocardial ischaemia and 2 hours reperfusion 24 hours later [18.8±3.6 vs 40.0 ±4.2% (p<0.01)] (unpublished observations). Moreover, it has been shown that the enhanced tolerance observed against lethal simulated ischaemia in neonatal rat cardiomyocytes 24 hours following ischaemic preconditioning, is abolished by pretreatment with the selective A_1 antagonist DPCPX [12]. These findings consistently suggest that transient adenosine A_1 receptor activation induces subacute myocardial adaptation resulting in delayed protection against myocardial infarction.

The adenosine receptor agonist used in our experiments, CCPA,

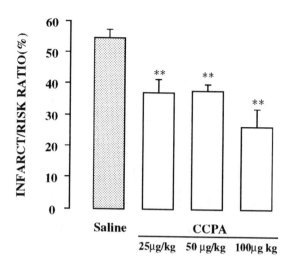

Figure 2. As a corollary of the experiment shown in figure 1, the effects of the selective adenosine A_1 receptor agonist CCPA was examined. Rabbits were treated with i.v. boluses of saline (filled column) or CCPA (open columns) and after 24 hours were subjected to an infarction protocol. Treatment with CCPA conferred significant limitation of infarct size, suggesting that transient adenosine A_1 receptor activation induces delayed myocardial protection 24 hours later. ** $P < 0.01$ vs saline (Dunnett's test). Adapted from Circulation 1994; 90: 2993-3000, with permission.

has a 10,000-fold selectivity for adenosine A_1 versus A_2 receptors and a subnanomolar affinity. It is therefore very likely that it is the transient activation of adenosine A_1 rather than A_2 receptors, that triggers delayed preconditioning against myocardial infarction. However, in our antagonist studies, SPT non-selectively inhibits adenosine receptors. Recent evidence suggests a role for adenosine A_3 receptors in mediating classic ischaemic preconditioning in the rabbit myocardium [13-15] and in isolated human atrial trabeculae [16]. We have not excluded a role for adenosine A_3 receptors in triggering delayed preconditioning and further studies are warranted to examine this issue.

Interestingly, no role has been demonstrated for adenosine receptors in the mechanism of delayed preconditioning against other endpoints of ischaemia-reperfusion injury. In conscious rabbits, the delayed protection afforded by ischaemic preconditioning against myocardial stunning following a subsequent period of ischaemia, is not abolished by pretreatment with non-selective adenosine receptor antagonists SPT or PD115199 [17]. Furthermore, transient adenosine A_1 receptor activation with CCPA fails to elicit delayed preconditioning against stunning in this model (see chapter 2). Similar results have been obtained in the pig myocardium [18] thereby excluding a role for adenosine receptors in the mechanisms of delayed preconditioning against stunning. Recent evidence from Bolli's laboratory has implicated a role for nitric oxide as both a trigger and a mediator of this form of protection. Similarly, nitric oxide seems to be involved in mediating the delayed cardioprotection against ventricular arrhythmias [19, 20], while the role of adenosine receptors in mediating this form of delayed protection has not been investigated (see chapter 4).

3. Time Course and Maintenance of Adenosine-induced Delayed Cardioprotection

In the next group of experiments we examined the time course of the delayed protection against myocardial infarction following transient adenosine A_1 receptor activation in our in vivo rabbit model [9]. Animals were treated with a single intravenous bolus of CCPA 100 µg/kg or saline vehicle. After a period of 24-96 hours the animals were subjected to 30 minutes coronary artery occlusion and 2 hours reperfusion and infarct size was assessed with TTC staining. CCPA treated animals had significantly smaller infarct size compared to saline treated controls at 24, 48 and 72 hours but no protection was observed at 96 hours (figure 3). The time course of protection after CCPA treatment in this model is identical to that of delayed cardioprotection following preconditioning with ischaemia previously reported by our group [21], and provides further evidence that adenosine A_1 receptor activation is an important physiological trigger of the delayed preconditioning phenomenon.

Although the anti-ischaemic effects observed during the 'second window of protection' following ischaemic or pharmacological preconditioning with CCPA are more sustained than that following the transient classic preconditioning phenomenon, in certain patient subgroups it may be desirable to extend the duration of this protection. Patients with unstable angina for example, are at high risk of death or myocardial infarction following an unstable episode and this risk is particularly high in the first 1-2 weeks [22]. These patients may therefore benefit from pretreatment with agents that trigger or augment myocardial preconditioning over a period of several days or weeks and could maintain the myocardium in a protected state.

Recent studies by Downey's group have addressed the possibility of extending the duration of classic preconditioning by using a continuous infusion of CCPA in a rabbit model of infarction (23). Rabbits subjected to a 6 hour infusion of CCPA showed a 59% reduction in infarct size compared to the saline treated group. Infarction in a group receiving a 72 hour infusion of CCPA however, was the same as in the 72 hour vehicle group. They concluded that myocytes become desensitised to the

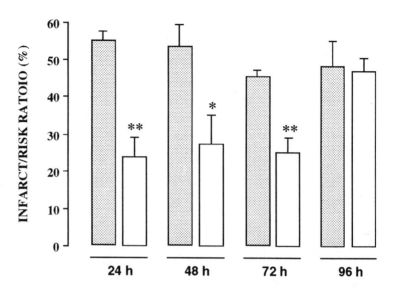

Figure 3. Time course of delayed protection induced by transient adenosine A_1 receptor activation. Saline (filled columns) or CCPA 100 μg/kg (open columns) was administered i.v. to rabbits. At the times indicated, they were subjected to myocardial infarction. Significant limitation of infarct size was observed at 24, 48 and 72 hours after CCPA treatment. * $P < 0.05$, ** $P < 0.01$ vs time-matched saline treated control group. Adapted from J Cardiovasc Pharmacol 1997; 29: 631-638 with permission.

protective effects of CCPA with prolonged exposure, and that such tachyphylaxis also abolished the beneficial effects of ischaemic preconditioning [23]. Similar results were obtained when they used repeated brief episodes of regional myocardial ischaemia as their preconditioning stimulus in a conscious, chronically instrumented rabbit model [24]. Animals subjected to 40 to 65 five-minute coronary occlusions over a 3 to 4 day period showed a marked attenuation in infarct size limitation compared to a group of animals that had been preconditioned with a single 5 minute occlusion.

The regulation of adenosine receptors has been studied in a number of different tissues and development of tachyphylaxis to adenosine A_1 receptors agonists has been shown to occur in a time- and dose-dependent manner [25, 26]. The time- and dose-dependence of A_1 receptor desensitisation would imply that reducing the dose-frequency of administering the agonist might delay the development of tolerance to its effects. We therefore hypothesised that the relatively prolonged nature of the protective effects of delayed preconditioning, as opposed to the short-lived classic preconditioning which only lasts for 1-2 hours following the preconditioning stimulus, may potentially allow "re-preconditioning" at 48-72 hour intervals, a time schedule that may maintain the myocardium

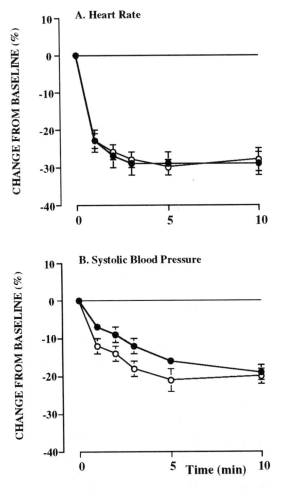

Figure 4. Haemodynamic responses to A_1 receptor activation after 10 days of intermittent CCPA administration. Rabbits were given i.v. boluses of saline (open circles) or CCPA 100 μg/kg (solid circles) every 48 hours. On day 10 they were subjected to an infarction protocol. Then, a further CCPA bolus was given to all animals. No differences in heart rate change or blood pressure change were seen in CCPA vs saline pretreated animals. Prolonged, intermittent dosing produces no tachyphylaxis. Reproduced from JACC 1998; 31: 1142-1149 with permission.

in a protected state without development of tolerance. To examine this possibility, experiments were performed during which rabbits were treated with repeated intravenous boluses of CCPA 100 μg/kg or saline at 48 hour intervals [10]. Forty eight hours after the fifth dose (day 10), the animals were anaesthetised and subjected to 30 minutes coronary occlusion followed by 120 minutes reperfusion. To further explore if the rabbits had developed tachyphylaxis to adenosine A_1 receptor activation, a subgroup of animals were treated with a further bolus of CCPA 100 µg/kg at the end of the reperfusion period and the haemodynamic response was monitored for 10 minutes prior to excision of the heart. Pretreatment with intermittent doses of CCPA resulted in a 42.0% reduction in infarct-to-risk ratio compared to vehicle pretreatment [26.6±3.7 vs 45.9±5.5% (P<0.01)]. Furthermore, CCPA treatment at the end of reperfusion resulted in identical hypotension and bradycardia in both groups implying no downregulation of A_1 receptor function (figure 4). Similar results have been obtained by another group using GR79236, a selective A_1 agonist which induced delayed protection at 24 and 48 hour in rabbits. Administration of GR79236 as a daily intravenous dose over a period of seven days resulted in the maintenance of protection which was evident 24 hours after the final dose [27]. These findings suggest that at least in the rabbit, the duration of delayed protection against infarction following pharmacological preconditioning with CCPA can be extended to a minimum of 10 days by intermittent dosing.

4. Signal Transduction Mechanisms

The signalling mechanisms downstream of adenosine A_1 receptors mediating its delayed cardioprotective effects are not completely understood and are currently under investigation. It has been shown that adenosine receptors may be linked to certain protein kinase C (PKC) isoenzymes via the diacylglycerol-phospholipase C pathway [28]. Furthermore, PKC seems to mediate delayed protection following ischaemic preconditioning in the rabbit heart [29]. On the other hand, one or more kinases in the mitogen activated protein kinase (MAPK) cascade, downstream of PKC, are activated by phosphorylation on tyrosine residues. For example, p38 MAPK requires dual phosphorylation on both a tyrosine and a threonine residue for its activation [30]. In addition, an important role has been demonstrated for tyrosine kinases in mediating delayed cardioprotection following ischaemic preconditioning [31]. We therefore examined the role of these kinases in mediating the delayed cardioprotective actions of adenosine A_1 receptor agonists [32]. Rabbits were treated with a bolus dose of CCPA 100 µg/kg or received saline. Prior inhibition of PKC with the specific antagonist chelerythrine chloride, or inhibition of tyrosine kinase with lavendustin A completely abolished the infarct limitation seen in CCPA treated animals after 24 hours (figure 5). Thus both groups of kinases play an essential role in mediating the delayed protection against infarction. The exact isoforms of PKC activated by CCPA are not known and their identification requires further investigation. Furthermore, the relative positions of PKC and tyrosine kinase in the signalling cascade downstream of A_1 receptors has not been elucidated. According to our results, since inhibition of either

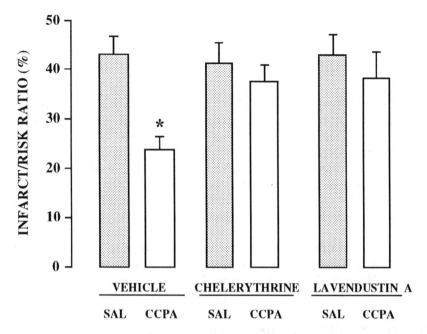

Figure 5. Involvement of both PKC activation and tyrosine phosphorylation in the delayed protective effects of A_1 receptor activation. Rabbits were treated with i.v. boluses of either saline (sal; filled columns) or CCPA 100 µg/kg (open columns). 10 minutes prior to these treatments, they received the PKC inhibitor chelerythrine hydrochloride (5 mg/kg), the tyrosine kinase inhibitor lavendustin A (1.34 mg/kg) or vehicle solution. After 24 hours, they were subjected to myocardial infarction. CCPA pretreatment induced delayed protection but this was abolished when either chelerythrine or lavendustin A were co-administered. * $P < 0.05$ vs corresponding saline treated group

enzyme completely abolishes the delayed protection induced by CCPA, it is likely that the enzymes are in series rather than in parallel pathways. Further details of the relative positions of these enzymes are currently under investigation in our laboratory.

5. Distal Mediator(s) of Adenosine-induced Delayed Protection

An important issue regarding the delayed protection against infarction conferred by transient adenosine A_1 receptor activation is the nature of the distal effector or target protein(s) that mediate this protection. The gradual onset and prolonged duration of protection following A_1 receptor activation is compatible with cellular mechanisms involving the new synthesis and degradation of cardioprotective protein(s). The exact nature of these protein(s) remains unknown. However, several hypotheses have been postulated and are currently under investigation in our and other laboratories.

Heat Shock Proteins

Heat shock or stress proteins (HSPs) represent a family of proteins which are induced or upregulated following a stressful stimulus such as hyperthermia, ischaemia-reperfusion or other oxidative stresses. Over the past few years, there has been great interest in the potential role of some of these stress induced cytoprotective proteins in mediating the delayed protective effects of ischaemic preconditioning (see chapter 7). We have investigated the regulation and localisation of a number of these HSPs many hours following pharmacological preconditioning of rabbits with CCPA.

Animals were treated with a single intravenous bolus of CCPA 100 µg/kg and hearts excised 24-72 hours later for analysis of HSP70i content by Western blotting. During this time course, no induction of HSP 70i was detectable suggesting that gross elevation of this protein is not the mechanism of CCPA-induced delayed protection [9]. In other studies, analysis of myocardial samples 24 hours after CCPA treatment did not reveal any changes in HSP70i, HSP90, HSP60 or HSP27 expression at the protein level [33]. On the other hand, subcellular fractionation studies showed a redistribution of HSP70i to the myofibrillar/nuclear fraction while HSP27 redistributed from the membrane to the soluble fraction. These results indicate that rather than changes in HSP gene expression, complex post-translational changes in HSP distribution may mediate the delayed adenosine induced cardioprotection.

Recent evidence indicates that adenosine treatment in perfused rat hearts results in rapid activation of MAP kinase-activated protein kinase-2 (MAPKAPK-2), a stress-sensitive kinase which is sequentially phosphorylated in a cascade of kinases involving p38 MAP kinase [34] (see chapter 5). HSP27 is one of the major substrates for MAPKAPK-2 and its phosphorylation has been suggested to play an important role in the regulation of actin microfilament dynamics [35, 36]. Furthermore, it has been demonstrated that increased expression of HSP27 in adult cardiac myocytes through an adenovirus vector-based approach results in enhanced resistance against injury mediated by stimulated ischaemia [37]. We therefore examined a potential role for post-translational modification of HSP27 in mediating adenosine induced delayed preconditioning [38]. Myocardial samples were obtained from rabbits pretreated 24 hours earlier with an intravenous bolus of CCPA 100 µg/kg. Two-dimensional gel electrophoresis and Western blotting of these samples revealed an acidic shift in the isoforms of HSP27 corresponding to an increase in mono- and bi-phosphorylated isoforms of HSP27 compared to hearts from saline

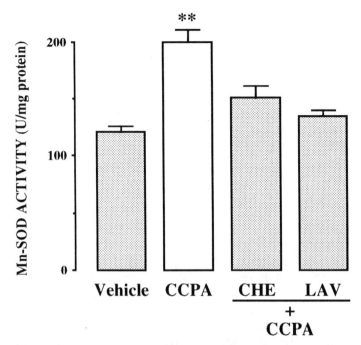

Figure 6. Modulation of endogenous antioxidant activity by transient adenonosine A_1 receptor activation. Rabbits were treated with either CCPA 100 µg/kg or a vehicle solution. Further animals were treated with CCPA preceded by injection of either chelerythrine chloride 5 mg/kg (che) or lavnedustin A 1.34 mg/kg (lav). After 24 hours, myocardial tissue was assayed for Mn-SOD activity using a colorimetric method. CCPA pretreatment significantly enhanced Mn-SOD activity in myocardium 24 hours later. This increase in antioxidant activity was abolished by either chelerythrine or lavendustin A. ** P < 0.01 vs vehicle.

treated animals. Furthermore, prior inhibition of either PKC or tyrosine kinase completely reversed this phosphorylation of HSP27. These results strongly suggest an important role for post-translational modification of HSP27 in mediating the delayed cardioprotective effects of CCPA although the exact relationship of these changes and the mechanism of protection remains unknown and requires further investigation.

Antioxidant Enzymes

Recent evidence suggests that one or more cellular antioxidant enzymes may be upregulated following heat stress or transient sublethal ischaemia and contribute to the cytoprotection observed during a subsequent lethal ischaemia-reperfusion injury (see chapter 8). One such enzyme which has received much interest in the past few years is the mitochondrial antioxidant manganese-superoxide dismutase (Mn-SOD). Yamashita et al. have recently reported induction of Mn-SOD induced by heat stress [39] or sublethal hypoxia [40] in neonatal rat cardiomyocytes at a time point that paralleled the delayed cytoprotection conferred by these preconditioning strategies. Moreover, treatment with antisense oligodeoxyribonucleotides corresponding to the initiation site of Mn-SOD translation inhibited the increase in Mn-SOD content and activity, and abolished the increased tolerance to hypoxia 24 hours after the preconditioning protocol. Recent reports indicate that treatment of a variety of tissues, including rat cardiac myocytes, with the adenosine A_1 receptor agonist N^6-(phenyl-2R-isopropyl)-adenosine (R-PIA) results in upregulation of a number of antioxidant enzymes including Mn-SOD over a 90-120 minute period [41]. We therefore examined a potential role for Mn-SOD in mediating the delayed cardioprotective effects of CCPA in rabbit myocardium [42]. Analysis of myocardial samples from animals pretreated 24 hours earlier with CCPA, revealed a significant increase in Mn-SOD activity compared to saline treated controls (200.3 ± 10.2 vs 120.3 ± 5.2 U/mg [P < 0.001]). Furthermore, this increase in Mn-SOD activity was attenuated by prior inhibition of either PKC or tyrosine kinase (figure 6), strategies that were also shown to abolish the cardioprotective effects of delayed preconditioning with CCPA. These results point to a possible role for Mn-SOD in mediating the delayed preconditioning effect of CCPA by reducing the reactive oxygen species induced injury during the index ischaemia-reperfusion. Further studies are ongoing in our laboratory in order to further characterise the role of these antioxidants.

K_{ATP} Channel

A wealth of evidence over the past few years has implicated a role for the ATP-dependent potassium channel (K_{ATP}) in mediating classic preconditioning in a variety of experimental models and species (reviewed in reference 43). The mechanism by which K_{ATP} channels exert this protective effect are not understood. It has been suggested that opening of sarcolemmal K_{ATP} channels results in a repolarising current that shortens the cardiac action potential thereby reducing the cellular calcium overload during the index ischaemia-reperfusion [44]. However recent evidence suggests that K_{ATP} channel openers may exert their cardioprotective effects without altering action potential duration [45]. This has prompted investigation into the role of K_{ATP} channels in other cell membranes such as the mitochondrial K_{ATP} channel in mediating ischaemic preconditioning. Diazoxide, a potent opener of mitochondrial K_{ATP} with weak actions on sarcolemmal K_{ATP}, has been shown to protect isolated rat hearts against ischaemic contracture and to improve post-ischaemic functional recovery [46]. These effects were shown to be independent of action potential duration and were reversed by K_{ATP} blockers glibenclamide and 5-hydroxydecanoate. Further studies are warranted to characterise the role of the mitochondrial K_{ATP} channel and the mechanisms by which it protects the ischaemic myocardium.

Delayed cardioprotection is induced by several adaptive stimuli. A number of studies have evaluated the role of K_{ATP} channels in mediating these subacute effects. For example, it has been shown that the delayed protection against infarction induced by heat stress is abolished by blockade of K_{ATP} channels in rabbit myocardium [47, 48]. Similarly, K_{ATP} channels have been shown to mediate delayed preconditioning against infarction induced by the endotoxin derivative monophosphoryl lipid A (MLA) [49, 50] (see chapter 9). Furthermore, some investigators have recently reported an important link between adenosine A_1 receptors and K_{ATP} channels in mediating the cardioprotective effects of ischaemic preconditioning. For example Randall et al. [51] and Cordeiro et al. [52] found enhanced response of the K_{ATP} channel to either ischaemia or a pharmacological opener of the channel in the presence of exogenous adenosine. Liu et al. have demonstrated a synergistic modulation of K_{ATP} currents by PKC and adenosine in isolated rabbit ventricular myocytes [53]. Furthermore, a recent study by Yao et al. has shown an important synergistic role between adenosine and K_{ATP} channels in acute memory of ischaemic preconditioning [54].

We therefore hypothesised that the delayed adaptive response to adenosine may also be mediated by K_{ATP} channels. In this respect, we have recently shown that blockade of K_{ATP} channels with either glibenclamide or 5-hydroxydecanoate prior to a long ischaemic insult, completely abolishes the protective effects of pharmacological preconditioning with CCPA 24 hours earlier in rabbit myocardium [55]. The mechanism by which transient activation of A_1 receptors result in subacute modulation of K_{ATP} channels is not known. The cellular localisation of the K_{ATP} channels mediating this delayed protection could conceivably be in the mitochondrion since 5-hydroxydecanoate is thought to be a modulator of mitochondrial K_{ATP} but not sarcolemmal K_{ATP}.

6. Conclusion

Adenosine is potent mediator of cardiovascular responses with actions on myocardium and conduction tissue, endothelium and vascular smooth muscle, and on the formed elements in blood. Adenosine is normally regarded as a short-acting mediator because it is rapidly deaminated or rephosphorylated. However, it is clear that in addition to acute effects, adenosine may also mediate sub-acute actions in myocardium, notably the induction of delayed tolerance to ischaemia-reperfusion injury. This sub-acute cardioprotective effect of adenosine appears to be an important component of the development of delayed ischaemic preconditioning in rabbit myocardium. Although in delayed preconditioning, effects of endogenous adenosine acting on A_2 and A_3 receptors at various sites can not be discounted at present, the sub-acute action of adenosine on myocardium can be mimicked by selective adenosine A_1 receptor agonists such as CCPA. The mechanisms by which adenosine A_1 receptor activation induces this late effect are not clearly understood but several possibilities have arisen including the regulation of HSPs, the upregulation of Mn-SOD and alterations in the opening characteristics of K_{ATP} channels, possibly on the mitochondrial inner membrane. The fact that this sub-acute cardioprotective action of A_1 receptor agonists is maintainable over prolonged periods suggests that this approach to protection of the ischaemic myocardium could have therapeutic potential.

Acknowledgements

The authors' work has been financially supported by the British Heart Foundation, the Medical Research Council of the United Kingdom, the Wellcome Trust and Glaxo-Wellcome. Dr Dana is supported by the British Heart Foundation through a personal (junior) fellowship and Dr Baxter is supported by a personal (intermediate) fellowship. The authors are grateful to Dr Nobu Yamashita for expert assistance in the assay of Mn-SOD.

References

1.   Mullane K, Bullough D. Harnessing an endogenous cardioprotective mechanism: cellular sources and sites of action of adenosine. J Mol Cell Cardiol 1995; 27: 1041-1054.

2.   Newby AC. Adenosine and the concept of "retaliatory metabolites". Trends Biochem Sci 1984; 9: 42-44.

3.   Moser GH, Schrader J, Deussen A. Turnover of adenosine in plasma of human and dog blood. Am J Physiol 1989; 256: C799-C806.

4.   Downey JM, Cohen MV, Ytrehus K, Liu Y. Cellular mechanisms in ischemic preconditioning: the role of adenosine and protein kinase C. Ann N Y Acad Sci 1994; 723: 82-98.

5.   Fisher S, Sharma HS, Karliczec GF, Schaper W. Expression of vascular permeability factor/vascular endothelial growth factor in pig cerebral microvascular endothelial cells and its upregulation by adenosine. Brain Res Mol Brain Res 1995; 28: 141-148.

6.   Giroud JP, Lian Chen Y, Le Vraux V, Chovelot-Moachon L. Activity of adenosine in relation to tumor necrosis factor (TNF). Therapeutic outlook. Bull Acad Natl Med 1995; 179: 79-99.

7.   Baxter GF, Marber MS, Patel VC, Yellon DM. Adenosine receptor involvement in a delayed phase of myocardial protection 24 hours after ischemic preconditioning. Circulation 1994; 90: 2993-3000.

8.   Marber MS, Latchman DS, Walker JM, Yellon DM. Cardiac stress protein elevation 24 hours after brief ischemia or heat stress is associated with resistance to myocardial infarction. Circulation 1993; 88: 1264-1272.

9.   Baxter GF, Yellon DM. Time course of delayed myocardial protection after tansient adenosine A_1 receptor activation in the rabbit. J Cardiovasc Pharmacol 1997; 29: 631-638.

10.   Dana A, Baxter GF, Walker JM, Yellon DM. Prolonging the delayed phase of myocardial protection: Repetitive adenosine A_1 receptor activation maintains rabbit myocardium in a preconditioned state. J Am Coll Cardiol 1998; 31: 1142-1149.

11.   Baxter GF, Kerac M, Zaman MJ, Yellon DM. Protection against global ischemia in the rabbit isolated heart 24 hours after transient adenosine A_1 receptor activation. Cardiovasc Drugs Ther 1997; 11: 83-85.

12.   Heads RJ, Latchman DS, Marber MS. Delayed preconditioning of neonatal rat cardiocytes by simulated ischaemia: investigation of A1-receptor, alpha-1-receptor and PKC involvement. Circulation 1997; 96 (suppl): I-313 (abstract).

13.   Armstrong S, Ganote CE. Adenosine receptor specificity in preconditioning of isolated rabbit cardiomyocytes: evidence of A_3 receptor involvement. Cardiovasc Res 1994; 28: 1049-1056.

14.   Armstrong S, Ganote CE. In vitro ischaemic preconditioning of isolated rabbit cardiomyocytes: effects of selective adenosine receptor blockade and calphostin C. Cardiovasc Res 1995; 29: 647-652 .

15.   Liu GS, Richards SC, Olsson RA, Mullane K, Walsh RS, Downey JM. Evidence that the adenosine A_3 receptor may mediate the protection afforded by preconditioning in the isolated rabbit heart. Cardiovasc Res 1994; 28: 1057-1061.

16.   Carr CS, Hill RJ, Masamune H, et al. Evidence for a role for both the adenosine A_1 and A_3 receptors in protection of isolated human atrial muscle against simulated ischaemia. Cardiovasc Res 1997; 36: 52-29.

17.   Maldonado C, Qiu Y, Tang XL, Cohen MV, Auchampach J, Bolli R. Role of adenosine receptors in late preconditioning against myocardial stunning in conscious rabbits. Am J Physiol 1997; 273: H1324-H1332.

18.   Sun JZ, Tang XL, Knowlton AA, Park SW, Qiu Y, Bolli R. Late preconditioning against myocardial stunning. An endogenous protective mechanism that confers resistance to postischemic dysfunction 24 h after brief ischemia in conscious pigs. J Clin Invest 1995; 95: 388-403.

19.   Kis A, Vegh A, Papp JG, Parratt JR. Pacing-induced delayed antiarrhytmic protection is attenuated by aminoguanidine in dogs. J Mol Cell Cardiol 1998; 30: A72 (abstract).

20.   Vegh A, Papp JG, Parratt JR. Prevention by dexamethasone of the marked antiarrhythmic effects of preconditioning induced 20 h after rapid cardiac pacing. Br J Pharmacol 1994; 113: 1081-1082.

21.   Baxter G, Goma F, Yellon D. Characterisation of the infarct-limiting effect of delayed preconditioning: time course and dose-dependency studies in rabbit myocardium. Basic Res Cardiol 1997; 92: 159-167.

22.   Williams DO, Brauwald E, Thompson B, Sharaf BL, Buller C, Knatterud GL. Results of percutaneous transluminal coronary angioplasty in unstable angina and non Q-wave myocardial infarction: Observations from the TIMI IIIB trial. Circulation 1996; 94: 2749-2755.

23.   Tsuchida A, Thompson R, Olsson RA, Downey JM. The anti-infarct effect of an adenosine A1-selective agonist is diminished after prolonged infusion as is the cardioprotective effect of ischaemic preconditioning in rabbit heart. J Mol Cell Cardiol 1994; 26: 303-311.

24.   Cohen MV, Yang XM, Downey JM. Conscious rabbits become tolerant to multiple episodes of ischemic preconditioning. Circ Res 1994; 74: 998-1004.

25.   Liang BT, Donovan LA. Differential desensitization of A_1 adenosine receptor-mediated inhibition of cardiac myocyte contractility and adenylate cyclase activity. Relation to the regulation of receptor affinity and density. Circ Res 1990; 67: 406-14.

26.   Ramkumar V, Olah ME, Jacobson KA, Stiles GL. Distinct pathways of desensitization of A1- and A2-adenosine receptors in DDT1 MF-2 cells. Mol Pharmacol 1991; 40: 639-647.

27.   Tavers A, Middlemiss D, Louttit JB. Cardioprotection after repeated dosing with GR79236, an adenosine A_1 receptor agonist. Br J Pharmacol 1998; 124 (proc suppl): in press (abstract).

28.   Gerwins P, Fredholm BB. Activation of adenosine A_1 and bradykinin receptors increases protein kinase C and phospholipase D activity in smooth muscle cells. Naunyn Schmiedebergs Arch Pharmacol 1995; 351: 186-93.

29.   Baxter GF, Goma FM, Yellon DM. Involvement of protein kinase C in the delayed cytoprotection following sublethal ischaemia in rabbit myocardium. Br J Pharmacol 1995; 115: 222-4.

30. Han J, Richter B, Li Z, Kravchenko VV, Ulevitch RJ. Molecular cloning of human p38 MAP kinase. Biochem Biophys Acta 1995; **1265**: 224-7.

31.   Imagawa J, Baxter G, Yellon D. Genistein, a tyrosine kinase inhibitor, blocks the "second window of protection" 48 h after ischemic preconditioning in the rabbit. J Mol Cell Cardiol 1997; 29: 1885-93.

32.   Dana A, Baxter GF, Yellon DM. Both protein kinase C and protein tyrosine kinase mediate adenosine induced delayed cardioprotection in rabbits. Circulation 1997; 96 (suppl): I-312 (abstract).

33.   Heads RJ, Baxter GF, Latchman DS, Marber MS, Yellon DM. Hsp and cytoskeletal protein expression and localisation during delayed preconditioning in the rabbit heart. J Mol Cell Cardiol 1998; 30: A20 (abstract).

34.   Kim SO, Salh B, Polech SL, Katz S. Activation of MAPKAP kinase-2 by adenosine in rat heart. Journal of NIH Research 1997; 9: 54.

35.   Guay J, Lambert H, Gingras-Breton G, Lavoie JN, Huot J. Regulation of actin filament dynamics by p38 map kinase-mediated phosphorylation of heat shock protein 27. J Cell Sci 1997; 110: 357-368.

36.   Benndorf R, Haye K, Ryazantsev S, Wieske M, Behlke J, Lutsch G. Phosphorylation and supramolecular organization of murine small heat shock protein HSP25 abolish its actin polymerization-inhibiting activity. J Biol Chem 1994; 269: 20780-20784.

37.   Martin JL, Mestrill R, Hilal-Dandan R, Brunton LL, Dillman WH. Small heat shock proteins and protection against ischemic injury in cardiac myocytes. Circulation 1997; 96: 4343-4348.

38.   Dana A, Skarli M, Yamashita N, Yellon DM. Delayed adenosine induced preconditioning: role of heat shock protein 27 and Mn-superoxide dismutase. Abstract submitted.

39.   Yamashita N, Hoshida S, Nishida M, et al. Heat shock-induced manganese superoxide dismutase enhances the tolerance of cardiac myocytes to hypoxia-reoxygenation injury. J Mol Cell Cardiol 1997; 29: 1805-13.

40.   Yamashita N, Nishida M, Hoshida S, et al. Induction of manganese superoxide dismutase in rat cardiac myocytes increases tolerance to hypoxia 24 hours after preconditioning. J Clin Invest 1994; 94: 2193-2199.

41.   Maggirwar SB, Dhanraj DN, Somani S, Ramkumar V. Adenosine acts as an endogenous activator of the cellular antioxidant defense system. Biochem Biophys Res Com 1994; 201: 508-515.

42.   Dana A, Yamashita N, Baxter GF, Yellon DM. Involvement of protein kinases and manganese-superoxide dismutase in adenosine induced delayed preconditioning. J Mol Cell Cardiol 1998; 30: A75 (abstract).

43.   Gross GJ, Mei DA, Schultz JJ, Mizumura T. Criteria for a mediator or effector of myocardial preconditioning: do K_{ATP} channels meet the requirements? Basic Res Cardiol 1996; 91: 31-34.

44.   Schulz R, Rose J, Heusch G. Involvement of activation of ATP-dependent potassium channels in ischemic preconditioning in swine. Am J Physiol 1994; 267: H1341-H1352.

45.   Yao Z, Gross G. Effects of K_{ATP} channel opener bimakalim on coronary blood flow, monophasic action potential duration, and infarct size in dogs. Circulation 1994; 89: 1769-1775.

46.   Garlid KD, Paucek P, Yarov-Yarovoy V, et al. Cardioprotective effects of diazoxide and its interaction with mitochondrial ATP-sensitive K^+ channels. Circ Res 1997;81:1072-82.

47.   Hoag JB, Qian YZ, Nayeem MA, D'Angelo M, Kukreja RC. ATP-sensitive potassium channel mediates delayed ischemic protection by heat stress in rabbit heart. Am J Physiol 1997; 273: H2458-H2464.

48.   Pell TJ, Yellon DM, Goodwin RW, Baxter GF. Myocardial ischemic tolerance following heat stress is abolished by ATP-sensitive potassium channel blockade. Cardiovasc Drugs Ther 1997; 11: 679-686.

49.   Elliot GT, Comerford ML, Smith JR, Zhao L. Myocardial ischemia/reperfusion protection using monophosphoryl lipid A is abrogated by the ATP-sensitive potassium channel blocker, glibenclamide. Cardiovasc Res 1996; 32: 1071-1080.

50.   Mei D, Elliot G, Gross G. K_{ATP} channels mediate late preconditioning against infarction produced by monophosphoryl lipid A. Am J Physiol 1996; 271: H2723-H2729.

51.   Randall MD, Ujiie H, Griffith TM. Modulation of vasodilation to levcromakalim by adenosine analogues in the rabbit ear: an explanation for hypoxic augmentation. Br J Pharmacol 1994; 112: 49-54.

52.   Cordeiro JM, Ferrier GR, Howlett SE. Effects of adenosine in simulated ischaemia and reperfusion in guinea pig ventricular myocytes. Am J Physiol 1995; 269: H121-9.

53.   Liu Y, Gao WD, O'Rourke B, Marban E. Synergistic modulation of ATP-sensitive K^+ current by protein kinase C and adenosine. Circ Res 1996; 78: 443-454.

54.   Yao Z, Mizumura T, Mei D, Gross GJ. K_{ATP} channels and memory of ischaemic preconditioning in dogs: synergism between adenosine and K_{ATP} channels. Am J Physiol 1997; 272: H334-H342.

55.   Baxter GF, Yellon DM. K_{ATP} channel blockade abolishes delayed anti-ischaemic actions of transient adenosine A_1 receptor activation. J Mol Cell Cardiol 1998; 30: A10 (abstract).

11

Angina and Cardiac Adaptation

F Ottani, M Galvani and D Ferrini

1. Introduction

Numerous studies have recently demonstrated that "preconditioning" the myocardium with brief episodes of coronary artery occlusion significantly reduces infarct size subsequently induced by prolonged occlusion. This phenomenon, termed "ischaemic preconditioning" [1] is the most powerful experimental method of delaying the onset of myocardial necrosis known so far, and its potent protective effects in the non-human heart are well established [2-4]. Of importance, the discovery has changed our perception of the consequences of myocardial ischaemia, and thereby of its major symptom, angina pectoris. In fact, angina, rather than always being harmful, may be regarded, in some specific clinical situations, as an indicator of increased myocardial resistance to lethal ischaemia [5-9]. In the clinical setting of acute coronary syndromes, and particularly of acute myocardial infarction (MI), the possibility that angina heralding MI may represent the clinical correlate of ischaemic preconditioning is extremely appealing because of its inherent cardioprotective action. Therefore, this chapter will review the concept that angina pectoris before MI may exert a protective role, through an adaptive preconditioning-like mechanism, and predispose to an improved post-MI prognosis.

2. Preinfarction Angina

By the middle of this century it was recognised that MI, previously considered a sudden clinical event, may be preceded by anginal episodes, especially at rest [10]. The term "preinfarction angina" was introduced to decribe this clinical situation. It is now clear that acute MI heralded by

Table 1. Theoretical human model of ischemic preconditioning derived from basic science experience.

Experimental features	Proposed human model
• BRIEF EPISODES (≥1) OF CORONARY OCCLUSION	• ANGINAL EPISODES (≥1) BEFORE INDEX MI
• REPERFUSION PERIOD AFTER PROLONGED OCCLUSION (optimal duration ≤ 180 min)	• REPERFUSION (≥ TIMI 2 FLOW) OF THE INFARCT-RELATED ARTERY IN A TIMELY FASHION (*ideally* maintaining the total time of prolonged ischemia ≤ 180 minutes)
• TIME-DEPENDENT RELATION BETWEEN PRECONDITIONING ISCHAEMIC EPISODES AND CARDIOPROTECTION EARLY PHASE (classic ischaemic preconditioning ; short-term effect, <2 hours) DELAYED PHASE (second window of protection, occurring ≈ 24 hours later)	• TIMELY-RELATED ONSET OF ANGINAL EPISODES TO MI (ideally <24 hours before index event) hours before MI → (classic or mixture of classic and delayed PC?) 12 to 24 hours before MI → ("pure" delayed form of PC ?)
• NO CORRELATION WITH COLLATERAL FLOW	• ABSENCE OF SIGNIFICANT EPICARDIAL COLLATERAL FLOW
END-POINT REDUCTION of INFARCT SIZE or correlates like global or regional LV function	END-POINTS REDUCTION of INFARCT SIZE or angiographic correlates like global or regional LV function *predisposing to* IMPROVEMENT OF POST-MI OUTCOME

prodromal attacks occurs with a rate ranging from 25 to 50% in different patient series [11-16]. Studies performed in the pre-thrombolytic era indicated that previous angina was associated with a higher baseline risk profile, as well as with an unfavourable clinical outcome [17-19]. These studies failed to observe any beneficial effects of preinfarction angina, although their interpretation is difficult in view of the absence of any reperfusion strategy. Reopening the occluded infarct-related artery is critical for preconditioning to occur. However, in the thrombolytic era, the widespread use of various reperfusion strategies has renewed interest in the protective role of preinfarction angina, as the clinical indicator of preconditioning.

3. From Experimental Laboratory to Humans

Although ischaemic preconditioning is a well-established phenomenon in the experimental laboratory, it should also be remembered that its capacity to limit infarct size in various animal models is strictly linked to the presence of a well-defined set of experimental characteristics. Unlike experimental scientists, who are able to control precisely experimental conditions, clinicians have to take into account many confounding variables that can easily obscure the occurrence of preconditioning in human infarcted heart. Thus, to overcome such difficulties it is necessary to devise an arbitrary human model of preconditioning, approximating as closely as possible to the experimental conditions, as summarised in table 1. The application of this template, which includes infarct-related artery reperfusion and onset of angina relatively shortly before MI, as well as demonstration of infarct size reduction, represents the first step to support the concept that preinfarction angina may precondition the human heart.

4. Pathophysiological Studies

Based on this pathophysiological background, there are only two studies [13, 14] that have reported infarct size reduction in patients with prodromal symptoms. Both studies included in their retrospective analysis patients with a first anterior MI treated with coronary thrombolysis or angioplasty largely within 6 hours from symptom onset. The timing of onset of anginal episodes, in our study [14], was limited to 24 hours prior to MI, while Nakagawa et al [13] extended the time-window to 1 week, even though 82% of patients complained of angina <24 hours before index MI. In our study [14] left ventriculogram analysis, performed 24 days after the index event to avoid myocardial stunning, showed a lesser number of hypokinetic segments in patients with prodromal angina (5.6 ± 4) compared with patients without angina (11 ± 7.5; P <0.04), despite a similar area at risk (figure 1). Based on such findings and excluding the presence of collaterals by protocol, ischaemic preconditioning was

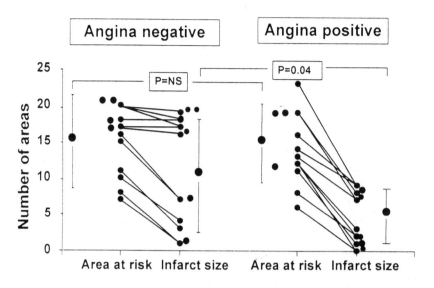

Figure 1. Final infarct size compared with area at risk assessed by ventriculography in patients with preinfarction angina <24 hours before MI and in patients without angina prior to index MI. Although a decrease in infarct size is shown in both groups, due to successful reperfusion of infarct-related artery, the reduction is significantly greater in patients with angina (69% vs 36%; P<0.05). This implies that the protective effect of preinfarction angina shortly before MI is of additional benefit to successul thrombolysis, as demonstrated by a further 33% reduction (95% C.I.: 7.1 to 58.9%) in the group with prodromal angina.

invoked as the mechanism underlying the observed reduction of infarct size. Nakagawa et al [13], reached similar conclusions using infarct-size correlates like global and regional LV function. By ventriculography repeated 4 weeks after the acute angiography, they showed (figure 2) a remarkably better recovery of ejection fraction in patients with prodromal symptoms compared with patients without angina; accordingly, regional wall motion was also improved (-2.72 ± 0.75 vs -3.14 ± 0.45 SD/chord, P<0.001), despite a similar initial damage (-3.34 SD/chord for both groups, P=NS). They also evaluated the role of collaterals by including a third group of patients with long-standing angina (>7 days). The global and regional LV function improvement detected in this group was mainly due to well-developed collaterals seen at baseline angiography (figure 2). In addition, after excluding patients with significant collateral flow, improvement of LV function parameters was detectable only in patients with prodromal angina (e.g. angina occurring 24 hours before index MI). Thus, besides the protection conferred by collateral flow, angina affords

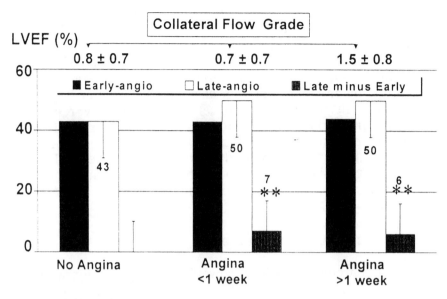

Figure 2. Global LV function changes in patients with preinfarction angina of different duration and in controls. Control patients (e.g., without angina) fail to show ejection fraction improvement between early and late angiography, while both groups with angina show a significant increase. However, the better LV function in patients with angina >7 days is due to the presence of large epicardial collaterals (collateral score:1.5 8, P < 0.05 vs the others two groups); whereas such condition does not apply for those with angina <7 days, who have a collateral score quite similar to patients without angina. These data show that, although collateral flow may afford some protection in patients with preinfarction angina, its beneficial effect can be visioned as adjuctive to another form of protection, which recognises preconditioning as the underlying mechanism.

cardioprotection per se through "preconditioning-like" mechanisms.

The clinical counterpart of the experimental observation that timely reperfusion is necessary for occurrence of protection conferred by preconditioning [1, 20] comes from the retrospective analysis of the MILIS study [21], a trial conducted in the prethrombolytic era, that observed a similar occurrence of in-hospital death, cardiogenic shock and congestive heart failure among patients with angina during the 3 weeks before MI as well as in those without angina. However, when considering only patients with spontaneous reperfusion of the infarct related artery as indicated by an early CKMB peak (<15 hours from symptom onset), patients with preinfarction angina showed a clear trend ($P = 0.09$) toward a smaller infarct size (10 vs 16 CK-MB gram-equivalent). On the contrary, patients without coronary reperfusion had similar infarct size, regardless of the presence or absence of prodromal angina. In summary, these data strongly suggest the occurrence of preconditioning in small and well-characterised patient populations. Additionally, in the presence of effective coronary reperfusion, preconditioning induces further reduction of infarct size (figure 1). Furthermore, preconditioning-induced myocardial salvage appears to be additional to the benefits conferred by collaterals (figure 2). Therefore, angina occurring shortly (<24 hours) before MI, namely prodromal angina, may represent the clinical marker of the experimental phenomenon.

5. Retrospective Clinical Studies

The logical consequence of such powerful cardioprotection would be a clear translation into better postinfarction outcome in patients with prodromal symptoms before MI compared with patients without angina. In the thrombolytic era, the simple retrospective analysis of large thrombolytic trials appeared to be an attractive and easy way to assess this issue having immediately available an adequate sample size to detect even small differences of clinical outcome, with confident statistical power.

Between 1992 and 1997, retrospective revision of 3 major thrombolytic trials were released, including TIMI IIb [22], the International Tissue Plasminogen Activator/Streptokinase Mortality Trial [23], and GUSTO-1 [24]. However, all studies, as summarised in table 2, failed to show any difference of post-MI outcome, or reported a worse prognosis in patients with previous angina. Both TIMI IIb [22] and the International Tissue Plasminogen Activator/Streptokinase Mortality Trial study [23], found a similar higher baseline risk profile in patients with angina. Furthermore, in TIMI IIb, Ruocco et al. [22] reported that patients with previous angina had more severe residual stenosis of the culprit vessel after thrombolysis (77% vs 73%, $p < 0.001$), more multivessel coronary artery disease and a higher rate of death and reinfarction than patients without angina. Barbash et al. [23] extended such observation to a 6-month follow-up, confirming a persistently higher mortality rate (14.8% vs 9.2%; p<0.0001) in patients with versus those without anginal symptoms. Also Migrino et al., recently reviewing the GUSTO-1 experience [24], found a negative association between previous angina pectoris and clinical outcome at 30-day follow-up: the overall 30 day mortality (6.8% vs 6%) as well as in-hospital cardiogenic shock and congestive heart failure were higher in patients with previous angina.

Such post-hoc analysis studies present many important drawbacks, which should be clearly pointed out. Although the appropriate timing of angina onset has been shown to be of fundamental importance, the inconsistent definition of preinfarction angina, with onset varying from <1 week up to 3 months before MI, might have strongly flawed the outcome results. Only Migrino et al. [24] have reported the occurrence of angina temporally related to index MI. However, probably due to the retrospective nature of the data collection derived from a multicentre clinical trial, the rate of patients complaining of chest pain 24 hours prior to MI was only 2.6%, unusually lower than the commonly reported 25 to 50% rate [7, 8, 10, 11]. Harper et al. [11] have demonstrated that the incidence of prodromal symptoms is higher when prospectively investigated by interviewing patients shortly after admission. Thus, only the prospective use of a specific questionnaire allows a detailed characterisation of the patients' symptoms, as we and others have reported [12, 14]. Finally, the absence of sufficiently detailed data on reperfusion of the infarct-related artery raises strong criticism against the results reached. Conflicting results, however, are reported by Muller et al. reviewing retrospectively the Thrombolysis and Angioplasty in Myocardial Infarction (TAMI) experience [25]. These authors found that previous angina, defined as recurrent chest pain beginning >7 days before infarction, favourably altered the in-hospital clinical outcome, despite the fact that patients with symptoms before MI exhibited a higher baseline risk, as reported in the quoted megatrials. Patients with angina showed a trend toward a lower in-hospital mortality rate (4.6% vs 7.2%). Among the possible explanations for this better short-term outcome in patients with previous angina, the investigators included preconditioning. It is, however, truly amazing to note that in the "no angina" group were also included patients with onset of angina <7 days. This subgroup of patients might have gained important protection by such anginal attacks occuring shortly before MI, thereby improving the overall clinical outcome in the "no angina" patients. Thus, the reported small difference of clinical outcome between patients with and those without previous angina in the TAMI study could have been somewhat lowered by this definition bias. In conclusion, all this retrospective body of data, far from clarifying the exact role of prodromal angina, i.e. chest pain of ischemic origin occurring within 24 hours prior to the index event, led to conflicting and confusing results. In our opinion, in light of the recent better characterisation of the preconditioning phenomenon [1-5, 28], this failure is mainly derived from the use of an incorrect model to study the phenomenon in the human heart (table 1). The crucial time-dependecy between the onset of prodromal angina and the protection afforded against the index MI is investigated in a totally inadequate fashion. Conversely, such studies clearly demonstrated that the longer the duration of antecedent angina, the higher the number of diseased vessels and, consequently, the worse the prognosis after MI (table 2).

An alternative line of clinical research applied more carefully the lesson derived from the basic laboratory to larger and less selected patient cohorts. Kloner et al. retrospectively evaluated the TIMI 4 trial patient population [12]; 155 patients had prodromal anginal attacks within 48 hours before index MI and 254 patients did not. The baseline characteristicts of both groups were nicely balanced, except for more frequent rate of multivessel disease (69% vs 57%; P = 0.02) in patients with prodromal angina. Effective reperfusion at 90 min angiography, defined as TIMI flow grade 2, was reached in the vast majority of patients of either group, with a trend (P = 0.11) to a higher reperfusion rate in patients with prodromal angina (81% vs 74%). Surprisingly, patients with angina were less likely to show collaterals than those without angina (9% vs 23%, respectively; p < 0.01). The study end-point was the combination of in-hospital death, cardiogenic shock and severe congestive heart failure, which was significantly lower (p<0.006) in patients with prodomal angina, as summarised in table 2. Of importance, cardiac death tended (P=0.09; table 2) to be lower in such patients, despite the relatively small sample size of the study. Furthermore, the retrospective analysis of a series of 350 patients with anterior MI recently published by Ishihara et al. [16] added impressive evidence supporting the protective role of prodromal angina. These authors found a significantly better (P<0.02) in-hospital survival in patients with prodromal angina, i.e. anginal attacks occurring within 24 hours, compared with patients without symptoms (table 2). In addition, this more favourable prognosis was maintained over a 5-year follow-up (86% vs 73% event-free survival; P<0.009).

6. Prospective Clinical Trials

The retrospective findings of better clinical outcome in patients with well characterised prodromal angina have laid the groundwork for prospective studies which are mandatory to confirm conclusively the previous observations. At the time of writing, however, only a few preliminary reports are available. Kloner et al. [15] have recently reported on the protective effect of prodromal angina occurring < 24 hour before index MI in the 3002 patients enrolled in the TIMI 9b trial. Patients with prodromal attacks had fewer cardiac events (i.e, combination of death, cardiogenic shock, congestive heart failure and recurrent infarction) compared with patients with angina of remote onset (i.e. >24 hours) or patients without angina (4% vs 14% and 12% respectively; P<0.02). Accordingly, such patients had lower peak CKMB release (1133 IU/L vs 1442 IU/L and 1570 IU/L respectively; P<0.01). A study performed by our group (26) tracks in the same direction of the TIMI 9b results [15].

Table 2. Effects of preinfarction angina on postinfarction outcome.

Large clinical trial post-hoc analysis

End-point	Trial	No angina	Angina	Time Course of Preinfarction angina		
	TIMI IIb	(n=1539)	(n=1798)	<7days (n=543)	8-180 days (n=516)	>180 days (n=736)
Death		4.0%	4.9%	6.1%	4.3%	4.5%
ReMI		4.6%	7.9%	9.0%	6.8%	8.0%
	Barbash	(n=4447)	(n=3882)	<1 Month (n=1.512)	>1 Month (n=2.370)	
Death		6.6%	10.8%	8.9%	12.1%	
ReMI		3.2%	4.6%	4.6%	4.6%	
	Gusto-1	(n=25740)	(n=13843)	<24 hours (n=1071)	>1-7 days (n=2491)	>7 days (n=10281)
Death		6.0%	6.8%	5.7%	6.5%	8.1%
ReMI		3.4%	5.9%	6.3%	4.6%	5.0%

Pathophysiologically-oriented clinical trials

End-point	Trial	No Angina	Angina
	TIMI-4	(n=254)	<48 hours (n=155)
Death		6%	3%
Death/Shock/CHF		10%	3%
	Ishihara	(n=261)	<24 hours (n=89)
Death		6%	14%

We have prospectively studied 417 patients with evolving MI, treated with thrombolysis; 40% of them had prodromal angina within 24 hours of MI. Both groups were balanced for baseline clinical characteristics. The rate of adverse in-hospital outcome (combination of death and cardiogenic shock and pulmonary oedema) was significantly lower among patients with angina as summarised in table 3. Furthermore, by Selvester electrocardiographic 32-point QRS scoring system [27], we also evaluated the ischaemic risk region (i.e. $QRS0$ score on the admission electrocardiogram) and the final infarct size (i.e. $QRS7$ score, on day-7 electrocardiogram after index MI). Although the analysis is still in progress, in the first 120 patients, despite a similar area at risk ($QRS0$ score: 12.5 ± 4.6 vs 13.0 ± 4.3; NS), those with prodromal attacks showed a trend toward smaller infarct size ($QRS7$ score: 5.2 ± 3.5 vs 6.4 ± 3.5; $P<0.1$). Thus, these preliminary results suggest that prodromal anginal attacks (<24 hours) before MI exert a protective role reducing infarct size and significantly improve post-MI prognosis. Furthermore, these investigations support the occurrence of cardioprotection through a preconditioning mechanism. However, many critical questions remain unanswered. Hopefully, they will be addressed when complete analysis of these studies is available.

Table 3. Prospective study of prodromal angina and in-hospital outcome in 417 patients with evolving MI treated with thrombolytic therapy

Endpoint	No Angina n = 252	Angina n=165	P
Death (n / %)	20 (7.9)	2 (1.2)	0.003
Cardiogenic shock	23 (9.1)	5 (3.0)	0.02
Pulmonary oedema	24 (9.5)	9 (5.5)	0.13
Combined *	33 (13.1)	10 (6.1)	0.02

*combined endpoint is a combination of cardiac death, cardiogenic shock and pulmonary oedema

It is well known that cardioprotection due to experimental preconditioning is critically time-dependent. This protective effect can be observed in two temporally distinct phases. An early phase, so called "classic" preconditioning, rapidly ensues after brief transient ischaemic episodes and is of short duration (< 2 hours). This is followed by a delayed phase, namely the "second window of protection", which occurs about 24 hours later [28]. Evidence for time dependence was recently suggested for patients with acute coronary syndromes, not elegible for thrombolysis, who underwent coronary angioplasty within 24 hour from the last spontaneous anginal episode [29]. It was, actually, found that the shorter the interval between the last spontaneous episode of angina and the initial balloon occlusion, the less evidence there was of an "ischaemic response", (i.e occurrence of chest pain and/or ST-segment shift). Nevertheless, as this interval increased, any naturally occurring preconditioning effect waned, substantially disappearing after 24 hours from the last anginal episode. In the setting of acute MI, the 24 hour time-window, taken as a whole, has been proven to exert an effective cardioprotection against lethal ischaemia; however, it is still unsettled whether a gradient of protection may exist within this time frame, with maximal benefit being present when preconditioning episodes occur within 6 hours prior to MI, as seen in unstable angina patients. Furthermore, whether or not anginal episodes occuring between 24 and 48 hours before MI are able to confer protection, as suggested by the retrospective data from TIMI 4, remains to be fully elucidated.

7. Preinfarction Angina: Is Preconditioning the Only Mechanism of Protection?

Collectively, the evidence presented so far allows us to propose that prodromal angina represents the clinical counterpart of ischaemic preconditioning. However, thrombotic occlusion of the coronary artery, which is the predominant cause of MI [30, 31], entails various important additional consequences. First, besides anterograde blood flow cessation, occlusion may acutely recruit collaterals [32], that could exert synergistic benefits with preconditioning in human infarcted heart [13]. However, the presence of epicardial collateral vessels is quite low (15% on average) in patients with a high rate of coronary reperfusion, and of similar incidence in patients with and without prodromal angina [12, 16, 24, 29]. Nevertheless, the impact of a collateral circulation remains incompletely disclosed until its possible relation between prodromal angina and opening of intramural and/or microscopic collaterals can be definitively assessed. Secondly, when thrombotic coronary occlusion is established, prompt reperfusion is crucial in reducing infarct size and preserving LV function [33, 34].

Recently, Andreotti et al. [35] reported, in a retrospective analysis of 25 patients treated with thrombolysis, that those with preinfarction angina of onset <1 week achieved more rapid coronary reperfusion than patients without angina. In fact, the difference in TIMI-3 flow rate was more pronounced earlier into thrombolysis in patients with angina than in

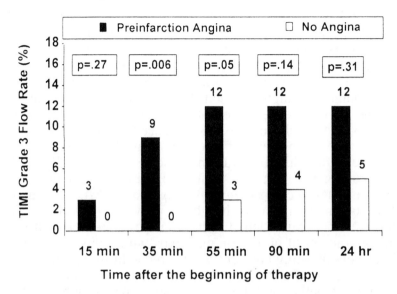

Figure 3. Rates of coronary reperfusion in patients with and without preinfartion angina. Angiography sequentially performed showed that complete reperfusion of the infarct-related artery (TIMI 3 flow) occurred very early into thrombolysis, being present at 35 minutes after the beginning of therapy in the vast majority of patients (9/14) with angina compared with patients without prodromal symptoms (0/8). The difference in the reperfusion rates between the two groups subsequently decreased over time.

patients without angina (figure 3), being already evident at 35 minute angiography in 64% of patients with a heralded MI. Accordingly, infarct size, estimated by enzyme release, was smaller than in patients without angina (102 IU/L vs 251 IU/L; P<0.03). The concept of more rapid thrombolysis is supported by Ishihara et al. [16], who recently reported a higher spontaneous rate of reperfusion in patients with prodromal (< 24 hours) angina than in those without symptoms (34% vs 22%, P=0.03). Furthermore, among patients who were given thrombolysis for an occluded artery, coronary reperfusion (TIMI 2-3 flow grade) was more frequently achieved in patients with prodromal angina (76% vs 56%, P=0.01), although the rate of complete reperfusion (TIMI 3 flow) did not differ between the "angina" patient and "no angina" patient cohort (64% vs 56%; P=0.18). However, the mechanism(s) by which an enhancement in thrombolysis occurs remains totally speculative at the present time.

8. Conclusion

Coronary artery occlusion caused by a fissured plaque with a superimposed thrombus, might be abrupt and lead to a sudden onset of MI without warning symptoms or, on the other hand, in a sizeable proportion of patients, there is an unstable phase in the hours/days preceding the complete arterial occlusion that manifests itself as transient myocardial ischaemia. This phenomenon, when symptomatic and temporally related (<24 hours) to evolving MI has now been shown to partially protect the tissue from the evolving necrosis [12, 14-16, 26]. At the same time, it is also possible that prodromal angina is not exactly synonymous with preconditioning as we know it from the basic laboratory. Several other mechanisms might be involved, such as collateral opening (intramural and/or microscopic channels) and more rapid thrombolysis [16, 35]. Of importance, a strict relation could exist particularly between preconditioning and prompt thrombolysis. Hata et al. [36] have recently demonstrated, in a dog-model, that release of adenosine caused by brief period of ischaemia preceding the longer occlusion may attenuate platelet aggregation, thereby contributing to facilitate the thrombolytic process.

Whatever the mechanism, it appears that patients with prodromal angina before MI exhibit, when rapidily reperfused, have a greater reduction of infarct size compared with patients without prodromal symptoms, and have a better post-MI outcome. At present, however, "optimal preconditioning–mimetic agents" are yet to be found, and "putting preconditioning in a bottle still remains a pharmacologic challenge" [37].

Acknowledgements

We are indebted to Francesca A. Nicolini, MD, PhD, for support and helpful criticism in improving the manuscript. We thank also Stefano Biancoli, MD for helping us in data handling.

References

1.   Murry CE, Jennings RB, Reimer KA. Preconditioning with ischemia: a delay of lethal cell injury in ischemic myocardium. Circulation 1986; 75: 1124-1136.

2.   Liu GS, Thorton J, VanWinlke DM, Stanley AWH, Olsson RA, Downey JM. Protection against infarction afforded by preconditioning is mediated by A1-adenosine receptors in the rabbit heart. Circulation 1991; 84: 350-356.

3.   Schott RJ, Rohmann S, Braun ER, Schaper W. Ischemic preconditioning reduces infarct size in swine myocardium. Circ Res 1990; 66: 1133-1144.

4.   Cohen MV, Liu GS, Downey JM. Preconditioning causes improved wall as well as smaller infarcts after transient coronary occlusion in rabbits. Circulation 1991; 84: 341-349.

5.   Deutsch E, Berger M, Kussmaul WG, Hirshfeld JW, Herrmann HC, Laskey WK. Adaptation to ischemia during percutaneous transluminal coronary angioplasty: clinical, hemodynamic, and metabolic features. Circulation 1990; 82: 2044-2051.

6.   Leesar MA, Stoddard M, Ahmed M, Broadbent J, Bolli R. Preconditioning human myocardium with adenosine during coronary angioplasty. Circulation 1997; 95: 2500-2507.

7.   Tomai F, Crea F, Gaspardone A, et al. Mechanisms of cardiac pain during coronary angioplasty. J Am Coll Cardiol 1993; 22: 1892-1896.

8.   Tomai F, Crea F, Gaspardone A, et al. Ischemic preconditioning during coronary angioplasty is prevented by glibenclamide, a selective ATP-sensitive K+ channel blocker. Circulation 1994; 90: 700-705.

9.   Yellon DM, Alkuhulaifi AM, Pugsley WB. Preconditioning the human myocardium. Lancet 1993; 342: 276-277.

10.   Mounsey P. Prodromal symptoms in myocardial infarction. Br Heart J 1951; 13: 215-226.

11.   Harper RW, Kennedy G, DeSanctis RW, Hutter AMJ. Incidence and pattern of angina prior to acute myocardial infarction: a study of 577 cases. Am Heart J 1979; 97: 178-183.

12.   Kloner RA, Shook T, Przyklenk K, et al. Previous angina alters in-hospital outcome in TIMI 4. A clinical correlate to preconditioning? Circulation 1995; 91: 37-45.

13.   Nakagawa Y, Ito H, Kitakaze M, et al. Effect of angina pectoris on myocardial protection in patients with reperfused anterior wall myocardial infarction: retrospective clinical evidence of "preconditioning". J Am Coll Cardiol 1995; 25: 1076-1083.

14.   Ottani F, Galvani M, Ferrini D, et al. Prodromal angina limits infarct size. A role for ischemic preconditioning. Circulation 1995; 91: 291-297.

15.   Kloner RA, Shook T, Antman EM, et al. A prospective analysis on the potential preconditioning effect of preinfarct angina in TIMI 9. Circulation 1996; 94 (suppl I): I-611 (abstract).

16.   Ishihara M, Sato H, Tateishi H, et al. Implications of prodromal angina in anterior wall acute myocardial infarction: acute angiographic findings and long-term prognosis. J Am Coll Cardiol 1997; 30: 70-975.

17.   Pierard LA, Dubois C, Smeets JP, Boland J, Carlier J, Kulbertus H. Prognostic significance of angina pectoris before first acute myocardial infarction. Am J Cardiol 1988; 61: 984-987.

18.   Cortina A, Ambrose JA, Prieto-Granada J. Left ventricular function after myocardial infarction: clinical and angiographic correlations. J Am Coll Cardiol 1985; 5: 619-624.

19.   Behar S, Reicher-Reiss H, Allmader E. The prognostic significance of angina pectoris preceding the occurrence of a first acute myocardial infarction in 4166 consecutive hospitalized patients. Am Heart J 1992; 123: 1481-1486.

20.   Ovize M, Kloner RA, Hale SL, Przyklenk K. Coronary cyclic flow variations "precondition" ischemic myocardium. Circulation 1992; 85: 779-789.

21.   Kloner RA, Muller J, Davis V. Effects of previous angina pectoris in patients with first acute myocardial infarction not receiving thrombolytics. Am J Cardiol 1995; 75: 615-617.

22.   Ruocco NA, Bergelson BA, Jacobs AK, Frederick MM, Faxon DP, Ryan TJ. Invasive versus conservative strategy after thrombolytic therapy for acute myocardial infarction in patients wirh antecedent angina. A report from Thrombolysis in Myocardial Infarction phase II study (TIMI II). J Am Coll Cardiol 1992; 20: 1445-1551.

23.   Barbash GI, White HD, Modan M, Van de Werf F. Antecedent angina pectoris predicts worse outcome after myocardial infarction in patients receiving thrombolytic therapy: experience gleaned from the International Tissue Plasminogen Activator/Streptokinase Mortality Trial. J Am Coll Cardiol 1992; 20: 6-41.

24.   Migrino RQ, Moliterno DJ, Topol EJ. Preinfarction angina (Letter). N Engl J Med 1996; 335: 59.

25.   Muller DW, Topol EJ, Califf RM, et al. Relatioship between antecedent angina pectoris and short-term prognosis after thrombolytc therapy for acute myocardial infarction. Am Heart J 1990; 119: 119-224.

26.   Ottani F. Clinical relevance of prodromal angina before acute myocardial infarction. "New concepts in acute coronary syndromes" 2nd International Meeting, Forlì, September 12-13,1997.

27.   Selvester RH, Wagner GS, Hindman NC. The Selvester QRS Scoring System for estimating myocardial infarct size. Arch Intern Med 1985; 145: 1877-1881.

28.   Yellon DM, Baxter GF. A "second window of protection" or delayed preconditioning phenomenon: future horizons for myocardial protection? J Mol Cell Cardiol 1995; 27: 1023-1034.

29.   Lim R, Laskey WK. Ischemic precondirioning in unstable coronary syndromes: evidence for time dependence. J Am Coll Cardiol 1997; 30: 1461-1465.

30.   DeWood MA, Spores J, Notske R. Prevalence of total coronary occlusion during the early hours of transmural myocardial infarction. N Engl J Med 1980; 303: 807-902.

31.   Davies MJ, Thomas AC. Thrombosis and acute coronary lesion in sudden ischemic death. N Engl J Med 1984; 310: 1137-1140.

32.   Sasayama S, Fujita M. Recent insight into coronary collateral circulation. Circulation 1992; 85: 1197-1201.

33.   Lincoff AM, Topol EJ. Illusion of reperfusion: does anyone achieve optimal reperfusion during acute myocardial infarction? Circulation 1993; 87: 1792-1805.

34.   The GUSTO Investigators. The effects of tissue plasminogen activator, streptokinase, or both on coronary-artery patency, ventricular function, and survival after acute myocardial infarction. N Engl J Med 1993; 329: 1615-1622.

35.   Andreotti F, Pasceri V, Hackett DR, Davies GJ, Haider AW, Maseri A. Preinfarction angina as a predictor of more rapid coronary thrombolysis in patients with acute myocardial infarction. N. Engl J Med 1996; 334: 7-12.

36.   Hata K, Kloner RA, Przyklenk K. The benefits of brief antecedent ischemia on platelet-mediated thrombosis are mimicked by brief intracoronary adenosine infusion. J Am Coll Cardiol 1997; 29: 179A (abstract).

37.   Cohen MV, Downey DM. Ischaemic Preconditioning: can the protection be bottled? Lancet 1993; 342: 6.

INDEX

INDEX

Developments in Cardiovascular Medicine

Developments in Cardiovascular Medicine

Previous volumes are still available

KLUWER ACADEMIC PUBLISHERS – DORDRECHT / BOSTON / LONDON

864340